# POST COVID-19 LONG HAULER

Frank Hamo
Post COVID-19 Long Hauler
Neurological Disorder



Published by BooxAI

ISBN: 978-965-578-133-5

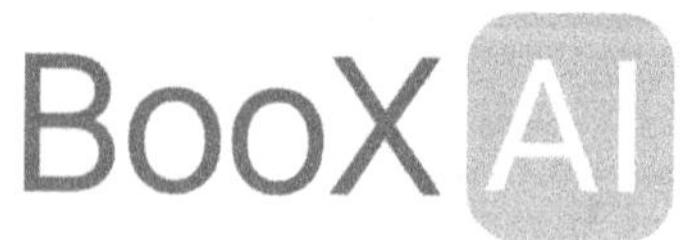

# POST COVID-19 LONG HAULER

## NEUROLOGICAL DISORDER

DR. FRANK HAMO

# CONTENTS

**1**

---

# BOOK EXECUTIVE SUMMARY

## 1.0 Book Executive Summary

Many people who have been sick with COVID-19, some who had mild or no symptoms, reported dealing with additional symptoms long after their acute illness ended. The long-haul COVID-19 symptoms can range from fatigue or headaches to mental health issues or chronic pain, involving multiple organ tissues damage due to the immune system cytokine storm response to the virus infection. It can ravage healthy cells during the process of fighting the infection.

Some people have been suffering for more than a year with no answers, no treatment options—not even a forecast of what the future may hold.

Researchers and data collection from scientists on post-COVID-19 illness had identified a few symptoms involving multiorgan symptoms as:

1. Brain neurological and limbic system COVID-related symptoms
2. Cardiovascular system COVID-related symptoms
3. Respiratory system COVID-related symptoms
4. Liver system COVID-related symptoms
5. Renal system COVID-related symptoms
6. Gastrointestinal system COVID-related symptoms

This book will concentrate on post-COVID-19 neurological disorders as a focus point by providing the patients with enough information on reported symptoms and detailed information about which parts of the brain are responsible for these symptoms.

**Note** these symptoms can be triggered by different factors other than post-COVID infection.

**This book will address screening and MRI diagnosis for the following symptoms as listed below. The provided samples of illustrated images are for informational and educational purposes only. Doctors can advise more images of diagnosis if required. Treatment options are beyond the scope of this book.**

*A- List of neurological disorder possibility results of post-COVID-19 infections or previous chronic conditions as listed below:*

1. Doing tasks in the wrong order
2. Finding difficulty to do multi tasks at the same time
3. Forgetting to do things often
4. Working on automatic, not thinking
5. Headache and getting tired after performing small tasks
6. Memory, concentration, or sleep problems
7. Depression or anxiety
8. Feeling tired or yawning all the time
9. Being more irritable than usual
10. Being frustrated by tasks
11. Having difficulty concentrating
12. Loss of smell
13. Vertigo

B- Introduction to brain anatomy

C- Brain modular lobe's function

D- Defining brain parts related to post-COVID-19 neurological dis- order symptoms

E- Imaging diagnosis for brain parts malfunctions using MRI technology

F- Brain modulars and neurons communication

Enhanced MRI Screening is advised to isolate the symptoms, physi- cian discretion is also advised.

**Note:** The symptoms that listed above can be caused by previous COVID infection as long hauler, or it can be caused by previous chronic illnesses. The purpose of this book is informational only for physicians and patients, and we do not provide solid evidence about this information. It is based on data collection from multiple clinical sources due to the fact most of these symptoms are still under clinical research and investigation.

**Treatment** option is beyond the scope of this book, and its physi- cian and specialist decisions come after performing a detailed and in-depth screening evaluation.

**Figure one: Brain Executive Functions**

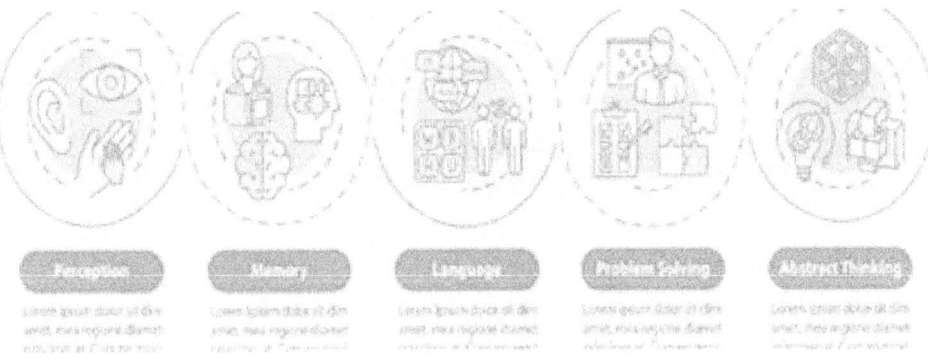

**2**

---

# BRAIN ANATOMY EDUCATIONAL INFORMATION

## 2.0 Brain Major Parts Anatomy

This section will provide the reader with enough information to understand the functions of the brain's main parts, including all four lobes. By comparing the parts' function and the manifestation of the post-COVID symptoms, it will make it easier for the reader to under- stand which brain parts are affected by the virus when discussing the symptoms with their physicians.

**Figure two: Brain anatomy showing four lobes, cerebellum, and spinal cord**

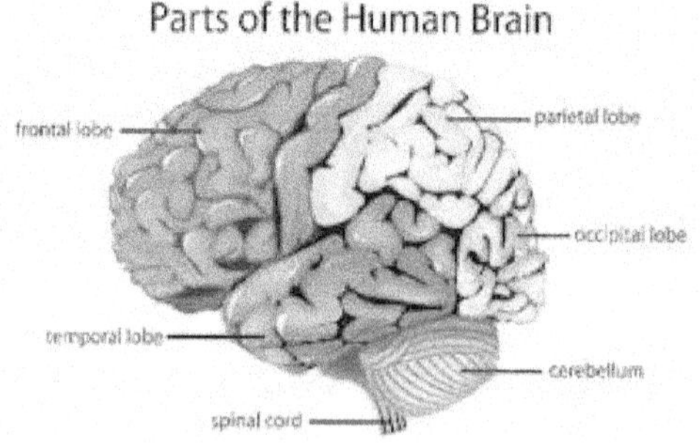

**The frontal lobes** are important for voluntary movement, expressive language, and for managing higher level executive functions.

## BRAIN ANATOMY EDUCATIONAL INFORMATION

**The temporal lobes** are also believed to play an important role in processing emotions, language, and certain aspects of visual perception, understanding language learning, and remembering verbal information.

**The occipital lobes** sit at the back of the head and are responsible for visual perception, including color, form, and motion. Damage to the occipital lobe will result in difficulty with identifying colors.

**The parietal lobes** are responsible for processing somatosensory information from the body; this includes touch, pain, and temperature.

**The cerebrum**, which forms the major portion of the brain, is divided into two major parts: the right and left cerebral hemispheres. The cerebrum is a term often used to describe the entire brain.

**Cerebellum** (which is Latin for "little brain") is a major structure of the hindbrain that is located near the brainstem. This part of the brain is responsible for coordinating voluntary movements, including motor skills such as balance, coordination, and posture.

**Brainstem** (or brain stem) is the posterior stalklike part of the brain that connects the cerebrum with the spinal cord. In the human brain, the brainstem is composed of the midbrain, the pons, and the medulla oblongata.

**Figure three: Brain High level Functions Illustration**

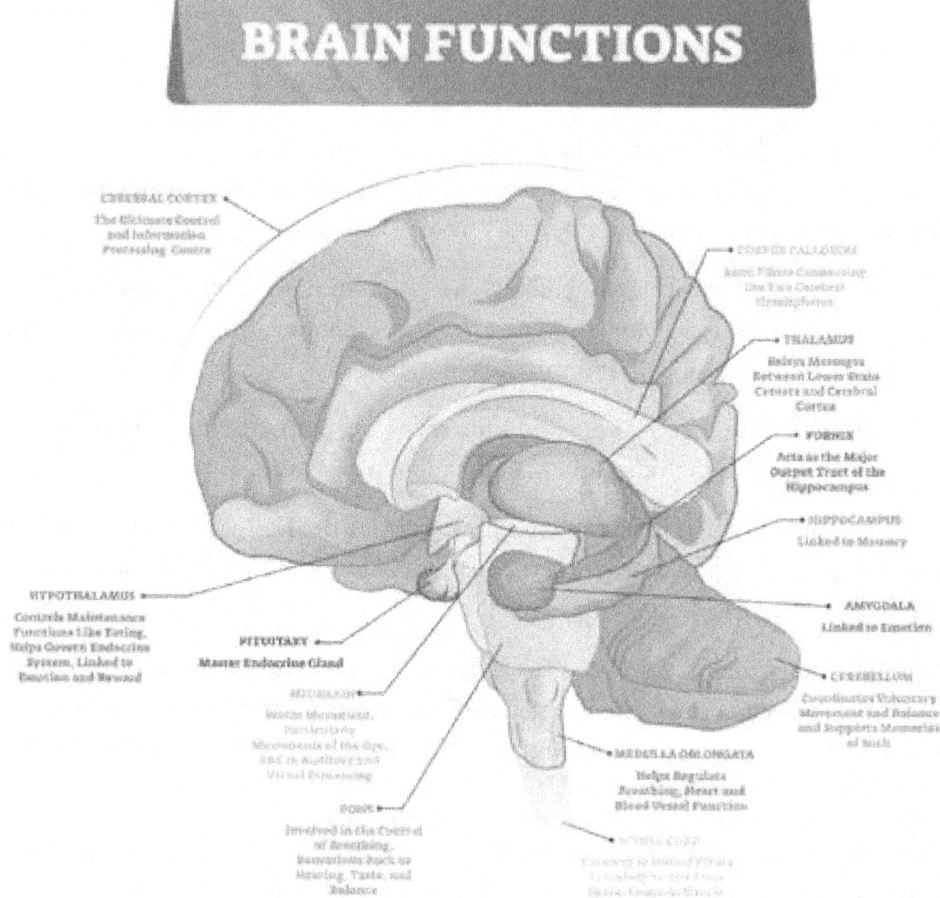

# Figure four: Brain High Level Four Lobes Functional Descriptions

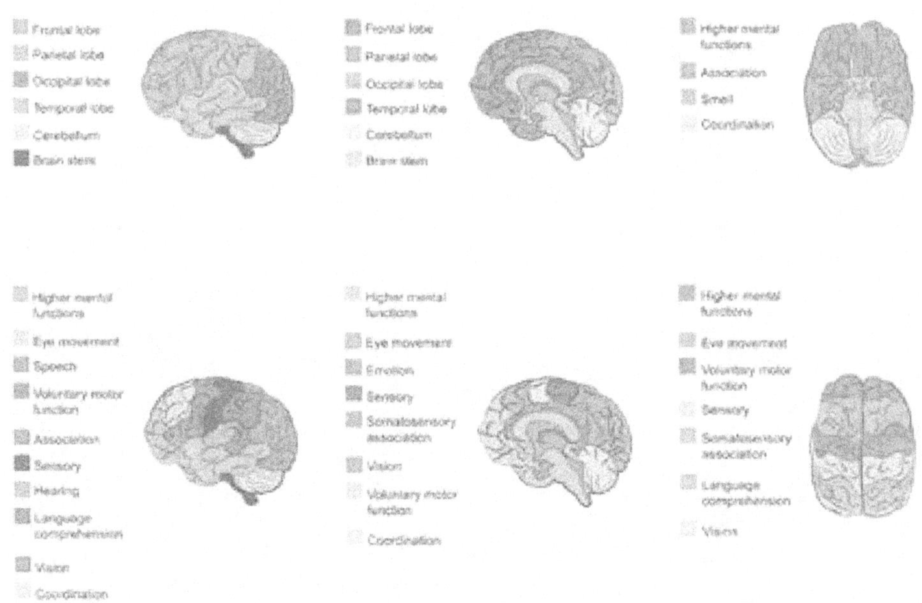

## 2.1 How Brain Communicates

Communication between neurons **occurs at tiny gaps called** synapses, where specialized parts of the two cells (i.e., the presynaptic and postsynaptic neurons) come within twenty to forty nanometers of one another to allow for chemical transmission.

### 2.1.1 How Brain Neuron Sends and Receives Messages

All the cells in our body communicate with each other. That is how we can do so many things in our daily lives: communication with each other by sending messages using a form of electricity. In neurons, this electricity is created by the flow of charged particles called ions, positively or negatively charged. The neuron has branches called dendrites, which send and receive signals.

Neuron communication junctions where vesicle fusion releases chemical signals are found at the end of axons.

**Figure five: How Brain Communicates**

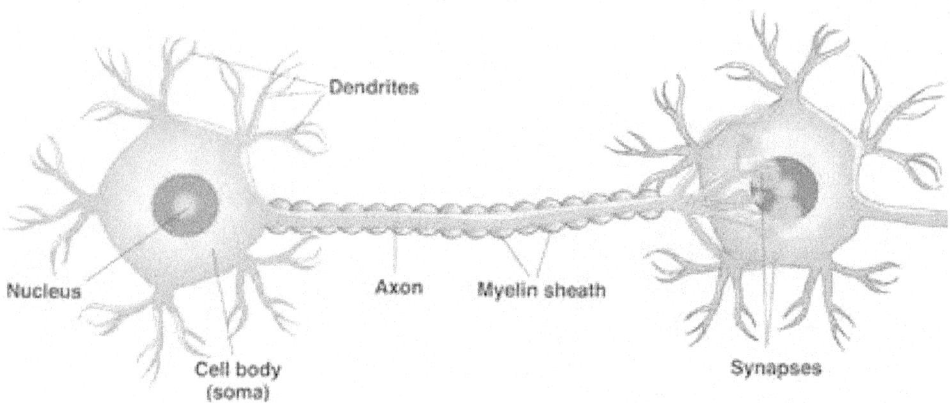


**Figure six: Brain parts responsible to performing tasks**

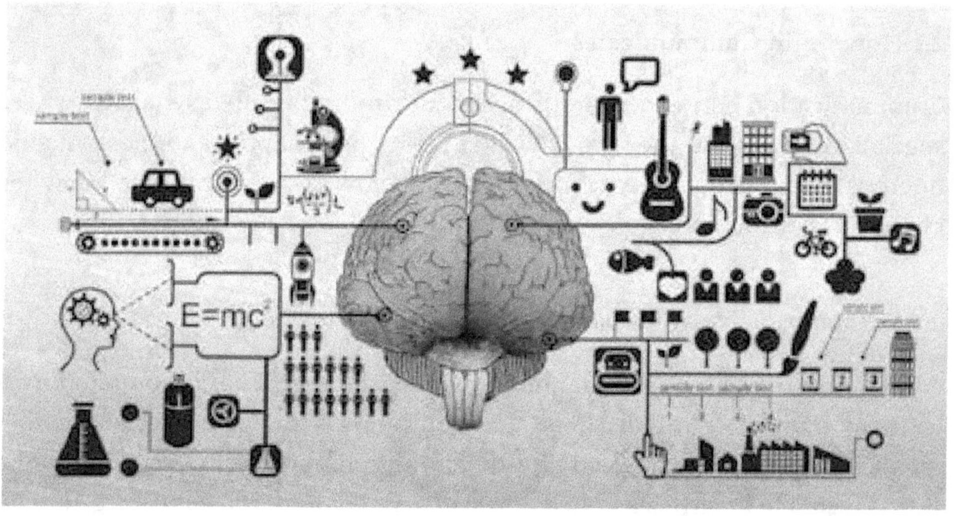

## 2.2 Human Brain Parts Functional Descriptions Overview

The brain is an amazing three-pound organ that controls all functions of the body, interprets information from the outside world, and embodies the essence of the mind and soul. Intelligence, creativity, emotion, and memory the brain is composed of the cerebrum, cere- bellum and brainstem.

*2.2.1 The central nervous system* (CNS) is composed of the brain and spinal cord. The peripheral nervous system (PNS) is composed of spinal nerves that branch from the spinal cord and cranial nerves that branch from the brain.

*2.2.2 Cerebrum* is the largest part of the brain and is composed of right and left hemispheres. It performs higher functions and fine control of movement.

*2.2.3 Cerebellum* is located under the cerebrum. Its function is to coordinate muscle movements, maintain posture and balance.

*2.2.4 Brainstem* acts as a relay center connecting the cerebrum and cerebellum to the spinal cord. It performs many automatic functions such as breathing, heart rate, body temperature, wake and sleep cycles, digestion, sneezing, coughing, vomiting, and swallowing.

*2.2.5 Right brain—left brain*

The cerebrum is divided into two halves: the right and left hemispheres. They are joined by a bundle of fibers called the corpus callosum that transmits messages from one side to the other. Functions of the hemispheres are shared. In general, the left hemisphere controls speech, comprehension, arithmetic, and writing. The right hemisphere controls creativity, spatial ability, art, and language in about 92 percent of people.

. . .

### 2.2.6 Lobes Functions of the brain

The cerebral hemispheres have distinct fissures, which divide the brain into lobes. Each hemisphere has four lobes: frontal, temporal, parietal, and occipital.

**Table one: Four Lobes Functions**

| Frontal lobe | Parietal lobe |
| --- | --- |
| Personality, behavior, emotions | Interprets language, words |
| Judgment, planning, problem solving | Sense of touch, pain, temperature |
| Speech: speaking and writing (Broca's area) | Interprets signals from vision, hearing, and memory |
| Body movement (motor strip) | **Temporal lobe** |
| Intelligence, concentration, self-awareness | Understanding language |
| **Occipital lobe** | Memory |
| Interprets vision (color, light, movement) | Hearing |
| | Sequencing and organization |

*2.2.7 CSF*

The cerebrospinal fluid (CSF) is **contained in the brain ventricles and the cranial and spinal subarachnoid spaces.** The means CSF volume is 150 ml, with 25 ml in the ventricles and 125 ml in sub-arachnoid spaces.

# Figure seven: Brain Lobes Functions Detailed Illustration

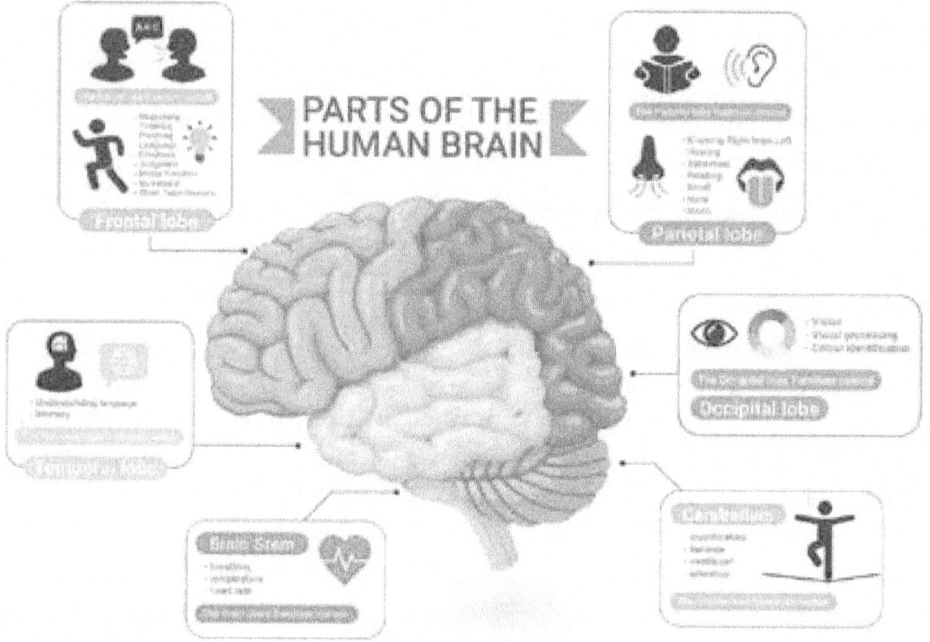



## 2.2.8 Cortex

The surface of the cerebrum is called the cortex. It has a folded appearance with hills and valleys. The cortex contains sixteen billion neurons (the cerebellum has seventy billion, which equals eighty-six billion total) that are arranged in specific layers.

## 2.2.9 Deep structures

Pathways called white matter tracts connect areas of the cortex to each other. Messages can travel from one gyrus to another, from one lobe to another, and from one side of the brain to the other.

.  .  .

*2.2.10 Limbic system concept* and human brain anatomy. **Basal ganglia, amygdala, thalamus, cingulate gyrus, and hypothalamus.** Below is a cerebral cortex and cerebellum medical infographic poster flat vector illustration. The Limbic system is the center of our emotions, learning, and memory.

**Gland Name:**

**Basal ganglia:** Function motor learning, executive functions and behaviors

**Amygdala Function:** Processing fearful and threatening stimulus

**Cingulate gyrus Function:** Helps regulate emotions and pain

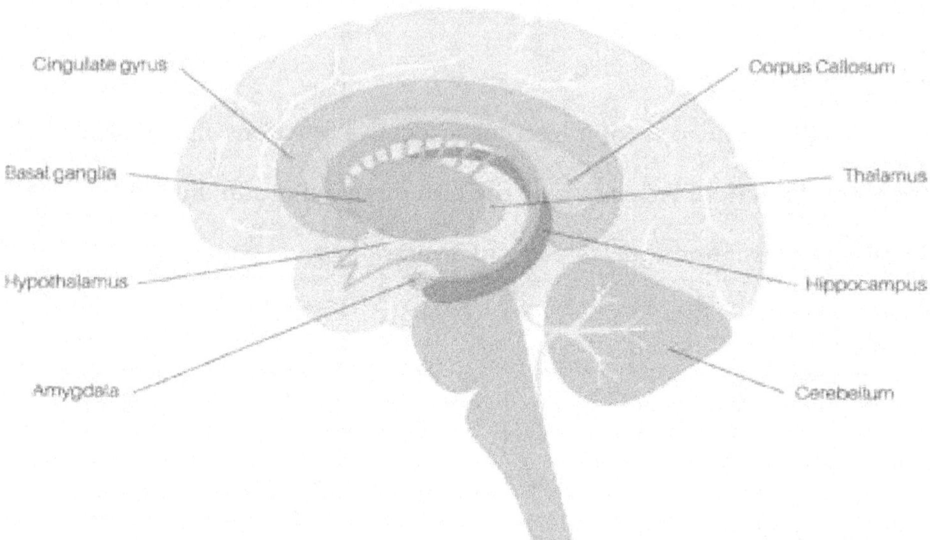


2.2.11 *Hypothalamus* is on the floor of the third ventricle and is the master control of the autonomic system. It plays a role in controlling behaviors such as hunger, thirst, sleep, and sexual response. It also regulates body temperature, blood pressure, emotions, and secretion of hormones.

2.2.12 *Pituitary gland* lies in a small pocket of bone at the skull base called the sella turcica. The pituitary gland is connected to the hypothalamus of the brain, known as the "master gland." It controls other endocrine glands in the body. It secretes hormones.

2.2.13 *Pineal gland* is located behind the third ventricle. It helps regulate the body's internal clock and circadian rhythms by secreting melatonin.

2.2.14 *Thalamus* serves as a relay station for almost all information that comes and goes to the cortex. It plays a role in pain sensation, attention, alertness, and memory.

2.2.15 *Basal ganglia* includes the caudate, putamen and globus pallidus. These nuclei work with the cerebellum to coordinate fine motions, such as fingertip movements.

2.2.16 *Cingulate gyrus* the cingulate gyrus helps regulate emotions and pain.

## 2.3 Brain Memory

Memory is a complex process that includes three phases: encoding (deciding what information is important), storing and recalling. Different areas of the brain are involved in different types of memory called encoding.

1. **Short-term memory** also called working memory, occurs in the **prefrontal cortex**. It stores information for about one minute, and its capacity is limited to about seven items.
2. **Long-term memory** is processed in the hippocampus of the **temporal lobe** and is activated when you want to memorize something for a longer time. This memory has unlimited content and duration capacity.
3. **Skill memory** is processed in the **cerebellum**, which relays information to the basal ganglia. It stores automatic learned memories like tying a shoe, playing an instrument, or riding a bike.

## 2.4 Ventricles and cerebrospinal fluid

The brain has hollow fluid-filled cavities called ventricles. Inside the ventricles is a ribbonlike structure called the choroid plexus fluid (CSF). flows within and around the brain and spinal cord to protect the brain from injury.

## 2.5 Cranial nerves

The brain communicates with the body through the spinal cord and twelve pairs of cranial nerves. The twelve pairs of cranial nerves that control hearing, eye movement, facial sensations, taste, swallowing and movement of the face, neck, shoulder, and tongue muscles originate in the brainstem. The cranial nerves for smell and vision originate in the cerebrum.

**Table two: Cranial Nerves**

| Cranial Nerve Name | Function |
| --- | --- |
| olfactory | smell |
| optic | sight |
| oculomotor | moves eye, pupil |
| trochlear | moves eye |
| trigeminal | face sensation |
| abducens | moves eye |
| facial | moves face, salivate |
| vestibulocochlear | hearing, balance |
| glossopharyngeal | taste, swallow |
| vagus | heart rate, digestion |
| accessory | moves head |
| hypoglossal | moves tongue |

## 2.6 Brain Blood supply

Blood is carried to the brain by two paired arteries, the internal carotid arteries and the vertebral arteries. The internal carotid arteries supply most of the cerebrum.

**Figure nine:** Brain Blood supplies

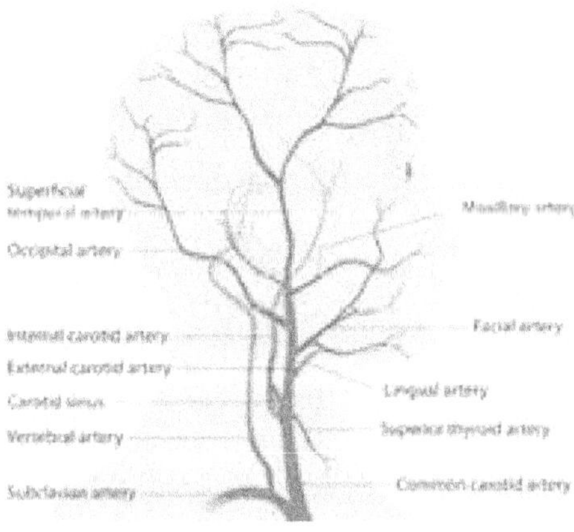

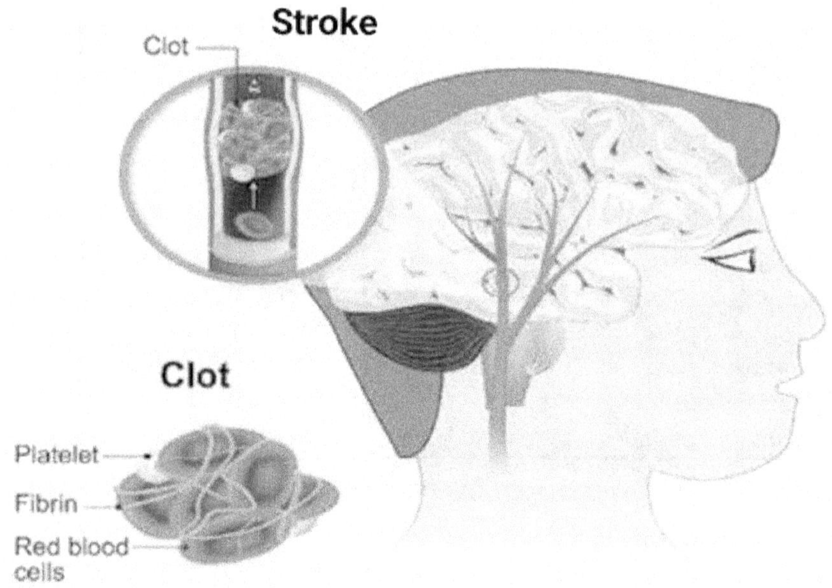


### 2.7 Brain Cells

The brain is made up of two types of cells: nerve cells (neurons) and glia cells.

### 2.7.1 Nerve cells

There are many sizes and shapes of neurons, but all consist of a cell body, dendrites, and an axon. The neuron conveys information through electrical and chemical signals. A neuron that is excited will transmit its energy to neurons within its vicinity.

### 2.7.2 Glia cells

Glia (Greek word meaning glue) are the cells of the brain that pro- vide neurons with nourishment, protection, and structural support. There are about ten to fifty times more glia than nerve cells.

Astroglia or astrocytes:

1. Oligodendroglia cells create a fatty substance called myelin that insulates axons, allowing electrical messages to travel faster.
2. Ependymal cells line the ventricles and secrete cerebrospi- nal fluid (CSF).
3. Microglia are the brain's immune cells, protecting it from invaders and cleaning up debris. They also prune synapses.

**Figure ten: Glial Cells Anatomy**

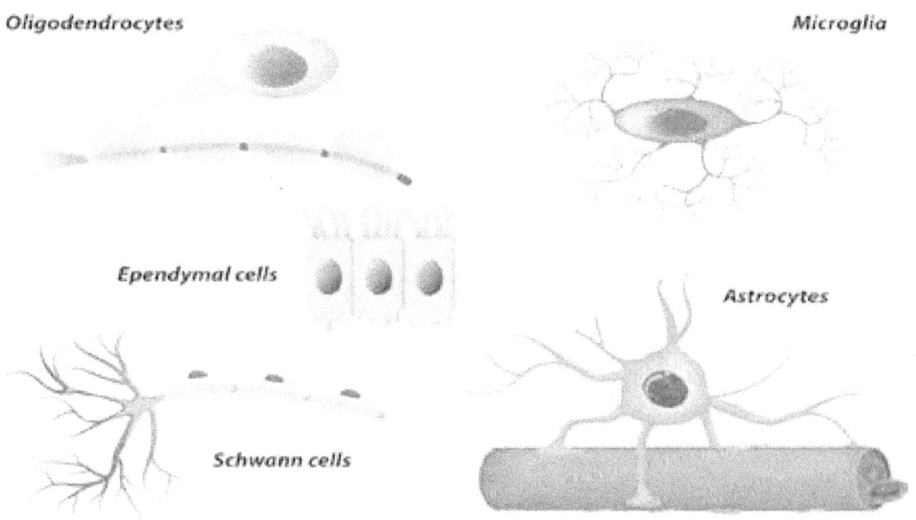

**3**

---

# DETAILED DESCRIPTION OF BRAIN COMMUNICATIONS

**3.0 Neurons are information messengers**

They use electrical impulses and chemical signals to transmit information between different areas of the brain and between the brain and the rest of the nervous system.

Neurons can only be seen using a microscope and can be split into three parts:

**3.1 Soma (cell body)**

This portion of the neuron receives information. It contains the cell's nucleus.

3.1.1 Dendrites: these thin filaments carry information from other neurons to the soma. They are the "input" part of the cell.

3.1.2 Axon: this long projection carries information from the soma and sends it off to other cells. This is the "output" part of the cell. It normally ends with several synapses connecting to the dendrites of other neurons.

·   ·   ·

3.1.3 Synapses are part of the circuit that connects sensory organs, like those that detect pain or touch, in the peripheral nervous system to the brain. Synapses connect neurons in the brain to neurons in the rest of the body and from those neurons to the muscles.

## 3.2 Memory may also involve the creation of new synapses

In the brain, the number and type of synapses are very dynamic. THERE are many ways that they are making behavior better; in other words, loss of synapses in the brain due to a degenerative disease, like Alzheimer's or Parkinson's, will cause a corresponding loss of function, but memory can recreate new synapses by improving and practicing remembering things.

### 3.2.1 Synapses

This electrical signal propagates like a wave along the long threads called axons that are part of the connections between neurons. When the signal reaches the end of an axon, it causes the release of chemical neurotransmitters into the synapse, a chemical junction between the axon tip and target neurons.

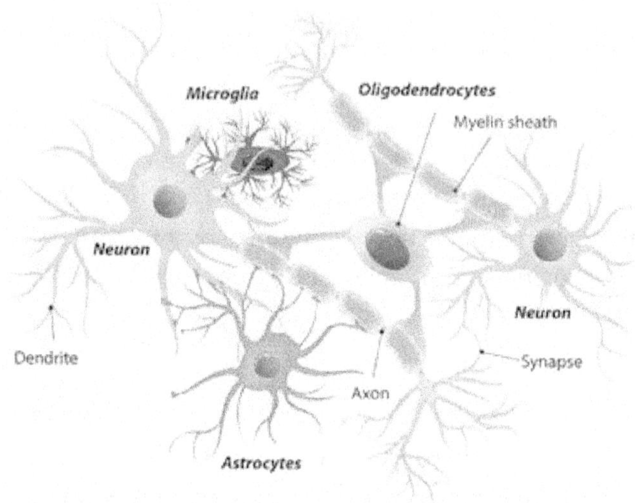



Neural communication. Transmission of the nerve signal between two neurons with axon and synapse. Close-up of a chemical synapse.

## 3.3 Deep Dive into Brain Internal Communication

3.3.1 Synapse, the electrical signal within the neuron is translated into the release of a chemical signal called neurotransmitter. Ions flowing into the axon terminal are the signal for vesicles containing neurotransmitters to fuse with the cell membrane to release neurotransmitters. The neurotransmitter then moves across to bind receptors in the receiving cell, which open to allow ions to flow into that cell, to perform certain function or task.

3.3.2 How does a synapse work to communicate between cells?

The electrical wave causes the neuron to release small chemical neurotransmitters at the synapse, which then travel across to the neuron on the other side of the synapse. This happens very quickly because the space is very, very narrow. When the chemical neurotransmitter reaches the receiving cell, it binds to a molecule called a receptor a membrane protein that binds the neurotransmitter to allow ion flow into the cell.

3.3.4 Synapses allow me to see and hear?

Our senses detect the world around us and transform the many external forms of energy (light, sound, movement) into electrical messages in our neurons. In our eyes, for example, there are light-detecting neurons that respond to the things we see. Some of these special neurons detect colored light (red, green, blue), and some detect just black and white. Light causes channels to open in light-detecting neurons, which sends an electrical message to the synapses of neurons inside your brain. This information is then processed by the brain to interpret the light images.

3.3.5 Many synapses communicate within the brain.

Seen image is an artist's rendition of neurons in your nervous system. The different colors represent the many different types of neurons, such as those that let you see and hear or learn and remember. The many projections from each neuron represent the many different synapses that neurons make with each other. The nervous system has a property called plasticity, which means that new synapses can form as we learn and strengthen as we make memories.

3.3.6 For us to hear, sensory receptors in our ears are activated by sound vibrations traveling through the air. These air vibrations move tiny hairs on the ear neurons. This movement opens channels, allowing ions to flood into the neuron and create the electrical message. As a result, neurotransmitters are released at the synapse between the hair cell and a brain neuron.

. . .

3.3.7 How do synapses allow me to learn and remember?

One of the most important things about our brains is that the number and size of synapses change when we use them. This property of the brain to change in response to what we experience is called plasticity.

The ability of all your synapses to change based on the amount you use them.

**Plasticity** allows us to learn new information and then remember what we have learned. If we use our synapses a lot, many more can form. If we do not use them as much, synapses can shrink or decrease in number. The strength of communication between synapses can also change depending on how much we use them, creating strong new synapses that remain in place for many years, even decades. This can help us to form long-term memories.

3.3.8 What happens when synapses do not work properly?

Since your synapses are so important for moving, sensing, learning, and remembering, it is easy to see how problems with synapses can cause diseases and disabilities. When synapses do not work properly, the brain cannot communicate within itself and with the muscles. Movement disorders often result from problems at the neuromuscular communication junction.

3.3.9 Why do we need to know about synapses?

So many functions of your body are carried out based on communication between cells that happens at synapses! Right now, as you are reading this, literally trillions of synapses are sending signals as zing around your brain and into the rest of your body. Neurons are driving movement in your muscles through neuromuscular junction synapses, allowing your eyes to move and your fingers to tap.

**Figure twelve: Synapse Anatomy**

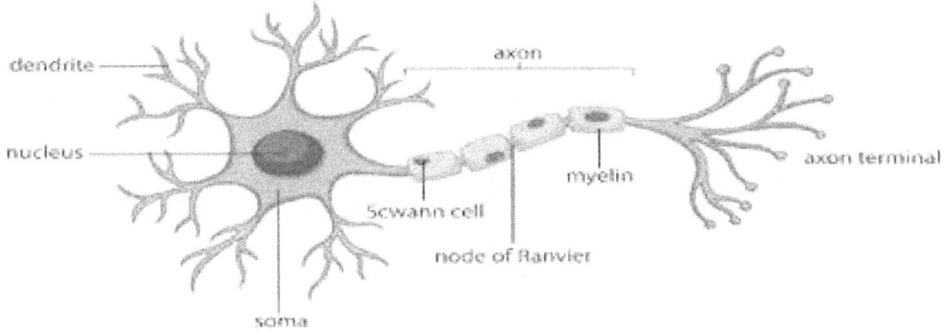



**Figure thirteen: Chemical Synapse**

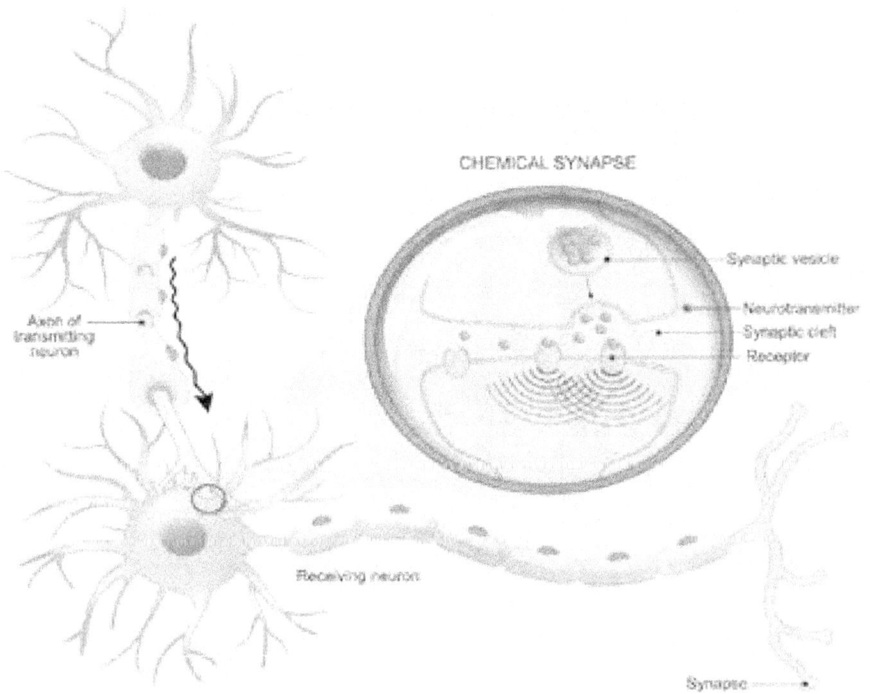

# 4

## HOW CORONAVIRUS INVADES BRAIN CELLS

**Figure fourteen: COVID-19 Proteins Structures**

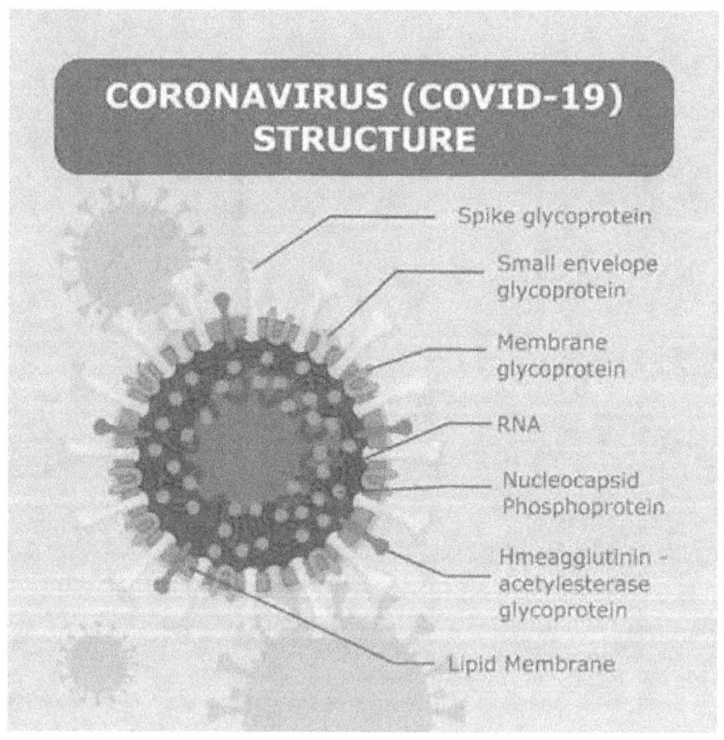

# 4.0 Virus genetic structure encodes four or five structural proteins:

S—spikes on the outside; mediates receptor binding

M—membrane protein; assists viral assembly

N—nucleocapsid protein; regulation of viral RNA synthesis, may interact with M protein during virus budding

E—small envelope protein; function necessary but not fully understood

HE—hemagglutinin-esterase glycoprotein

## 4.1 COVID-19 Brain Invasion Through Olfactory Explained

One way in which SARS-CoV-2 might be accessing the brain, experts say, is **by passing through the olfactory mucosa, the lining of the nasal cavity, which borders the brain.** The virus is often found in the nasal cavity—one reason that healthcare workers test for COVID-19 by swabbing the nose.

Researcher studies now suggest that SARS-CoV-2 can infect astrocytes, a type of cell that's abundant in the brain and has many functions. "Astrocytes do quite a lot that supports normal brain function," including providing nutrients to neurons to keep them working. Functions of astrocytes include **physical and metabolic support for neurons,** detoxification, guidance during migration, regulation of energy metabolism, electrical insulation (for unmyelinated axons), transport of blood-borne material to the neuron, and reaction to injury.

Study shows evidence of SARS-CoV-2 infection, 66 percent of the affected cells were **Astrocytes.**

Astrocytes are non-neuronal cells that regulate synapses, neuronal circuits.

### 4.1.1 Where Brain Astrocytes Cells Can Be Found

Neurons coexist with other types of cells in the central nervous sys- tem, such as **microglia** and **astrocytes.** According to cell-type distri- bution analysis, nuclear expression of ACE2 was found in many neu- rons (both excitatory and inhibitory neurons) and some non-neuron cells (mainly **astrocytes, oligoden-drocytes, and endothelial cells** in the human middle temporal gyrus and posterior cingulate cortex). This high expression of **ACE2** in **astrocytes** and some **neurons** is mainly located below the principal cell layers of CA1 and CA2.

4.1.2 Astrocytes Cells Function

Functions of astrocytes include physical and metabolic support for neurons, detoxification, guidance during migration, regulation of energy metabolism, **electrical insulation** (for unmyelinated axons), transport of blood-borne material to the neuron, and reaction to injury.

SARS-CoV-2 does not travel along the olfactory nerve, but it can reach the brain via the cranial nerve that runs close to the olfactory nerve into the brain: the nervus terminalis. This little-known cranial nerve connects the olfactory epithelium directly with brain structures cau- dal to the olfactory bulb.

A major fraction of the neurons in the nervus terminalis express the virus entry protein ACE2. Since this cranial nerve connects the olfac- tory epithelium directly with the hypothalamus, that concluded that the nervus terminalis may provide a route for the virus to reach the brain.

Hypothalamus, bypassing the olfactory bulb. Once virus reaches the hypothalamus, SARS-CoV-2 can penetrate the blood-brain-bar- rier and can reach various neural circuits connected to the hypo- thalamus, including brain-stem nuclei that are involved in respira- tion. Interestingly, the hypothalamus and the choroid plexus express ACE2, and this may provide a basis for dysfunction of the renin-angiotensin system (RAS) and blood pressure dysregulation, especially in elderly COVID patients who have a compromised RAS due to aging and who are particularly at risk for severe COVID-19.

**In nutshell:** Brain neurological symptoms are caused by COVID-19 infection of Astrocytes and Glia cells as results. Synapse proximity can be damaged or altered and cause numbers of neurological symptoms. The synapses communicate with each other at close proximity of 20–40 nm.

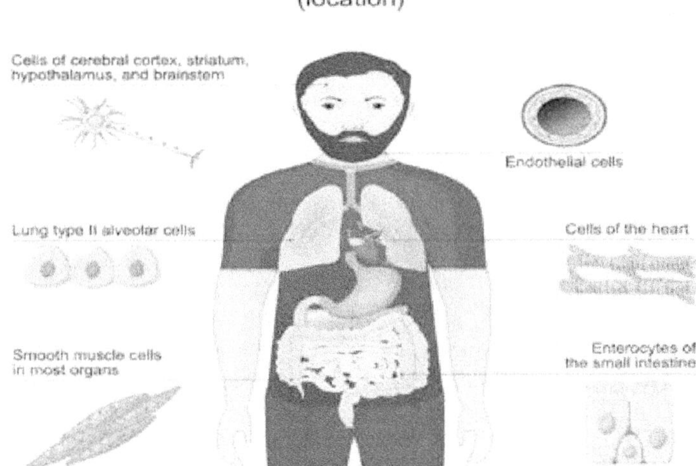



**Figure fifteen: Astrocytes Cell Anatomy Illustration**

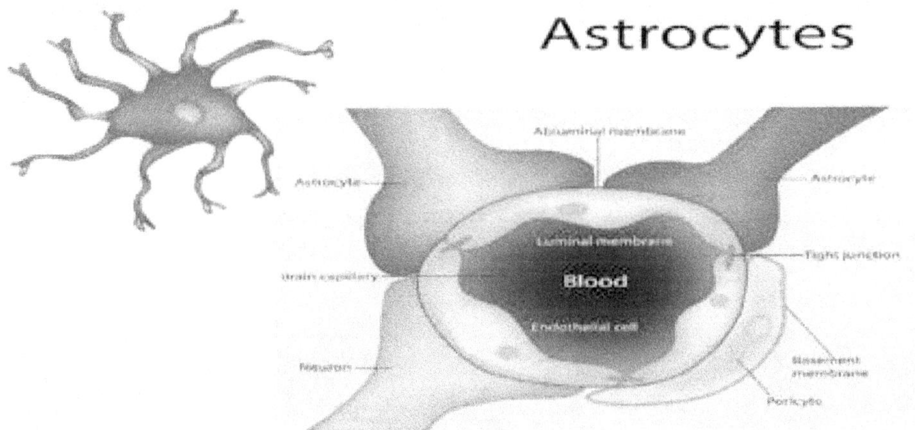

**Figure sixteen: Olfactory Nerve Anatomy**

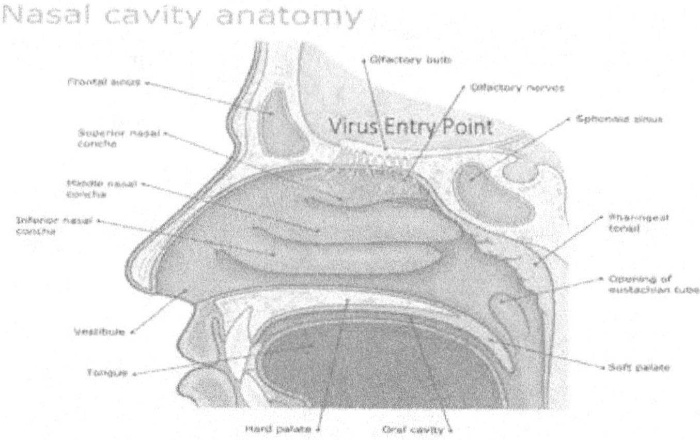


**Figure seventeen: Olfactory Cells**

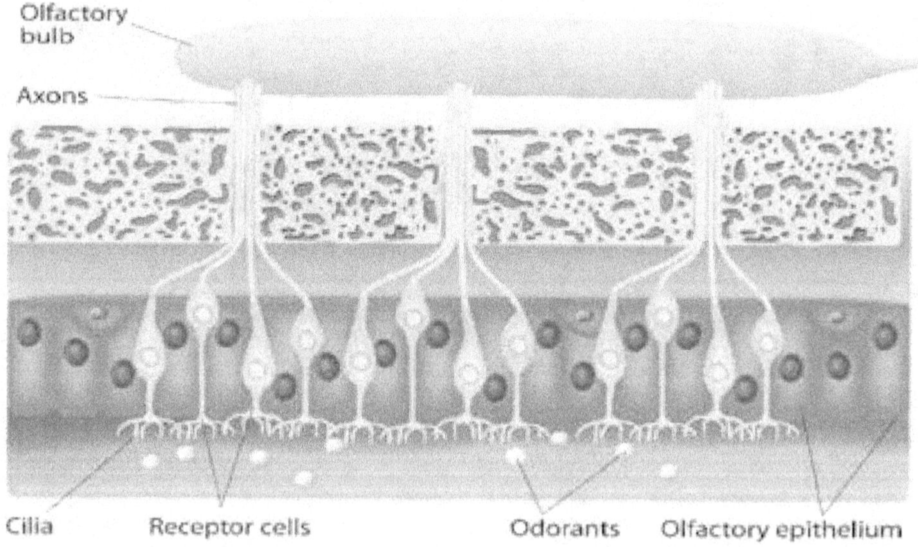

**Figure eighteen: Olfactory Physical Location Illustration**

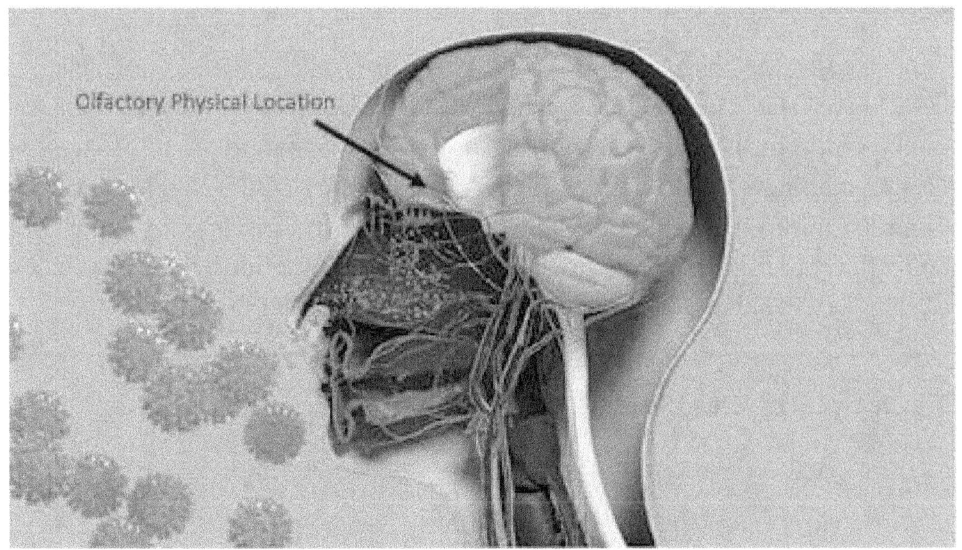


**Figure ninteen: Olfactory Location Near Thalamus Illustration**

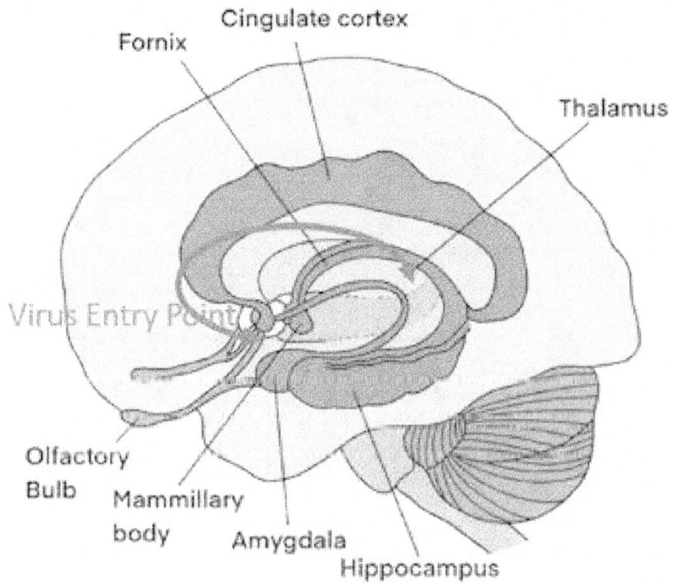

## 4.2 COVID-19 Brain Invasion Through Lungs Capillary and Blood Flow Explained

During infection with a severe acute respiratory syndrome, corona- virus 2 (SARS-CoV-2) in humans is associated with a broad spectrum of clinical respiratory syndromes, ranging from mild upper airway symptoms to progressive life-threatening viral pneumonia. Clinically, patients with severe coronavirus disease 2019 (COVID- 19) have labored breathing and progressive hypoxemia and often receive mechanical ventilatory. A virus may escape to the blood stream via a capillary vein and endothelial cells and reach the brain.

**Figure twenty: Virus Escapes from Alveoli**

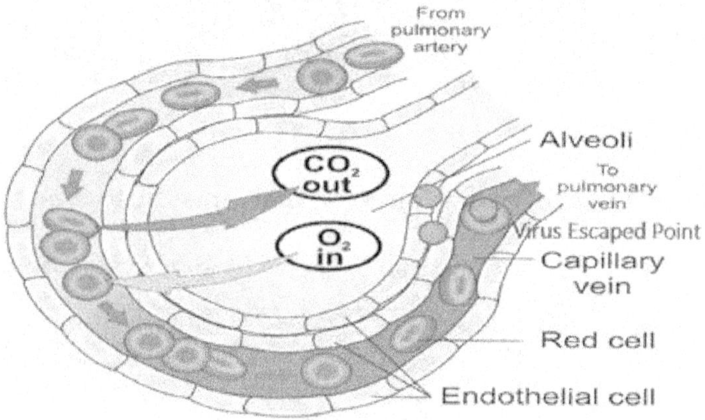


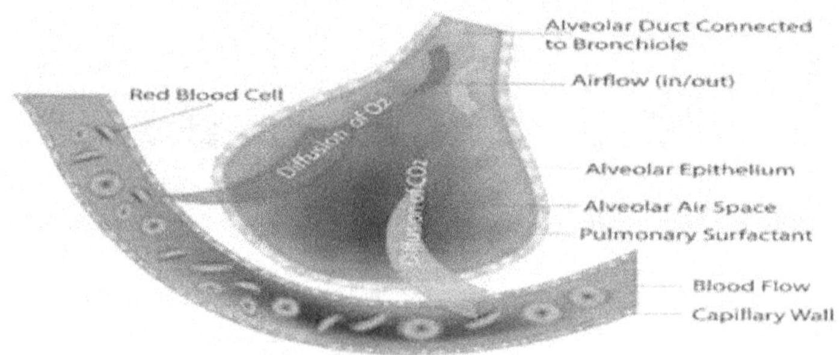

## 4.3 Brain Blood Brain Barrier

The purpose of the blood brain barrier is **to protect against**

**circulating toxins or pathogens that could cause brain infections.** COVID-19 virus can enter the brain through brain blood barrier.

**Figure twenty-one: Brain Blood Barrier**

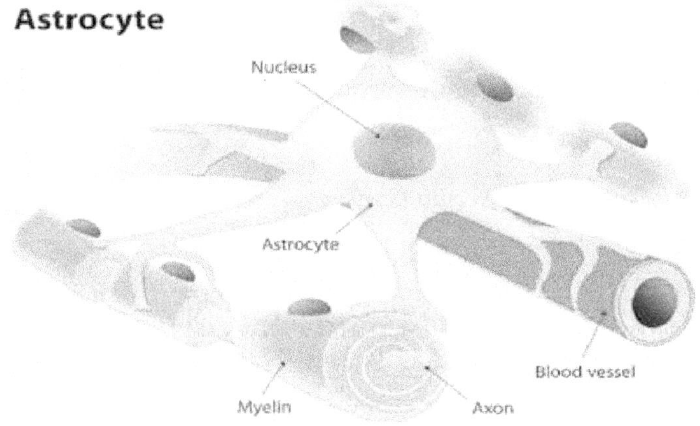


**Figure twenty-two: Brain Blood Barrier under Electron Microscope**

Showing Damaged Astrocyte as results of prior COVID infection

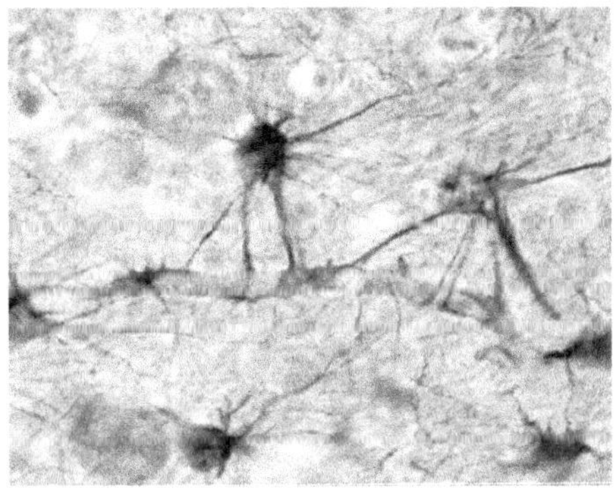

## 4.4 COVID virus was detected in brain tissues

Neurological complications are common in COVID-19. Although SARS-CoV-2 has been detected in patients' brain tissues, its entry routes and resulting consequences are not well understood. Here, we show a pronounced upregulation of interferon signaling pathways of the neurovascular unit in fatal COVID-19, by investigating the susceptibility of human induced pluripotent stem cell (hiPSC)-de- rived brain capillary endothelial-like cells (BCECs) to SARS-CoV-2 infection.

**Figure twenty-three: Inter Neurons**

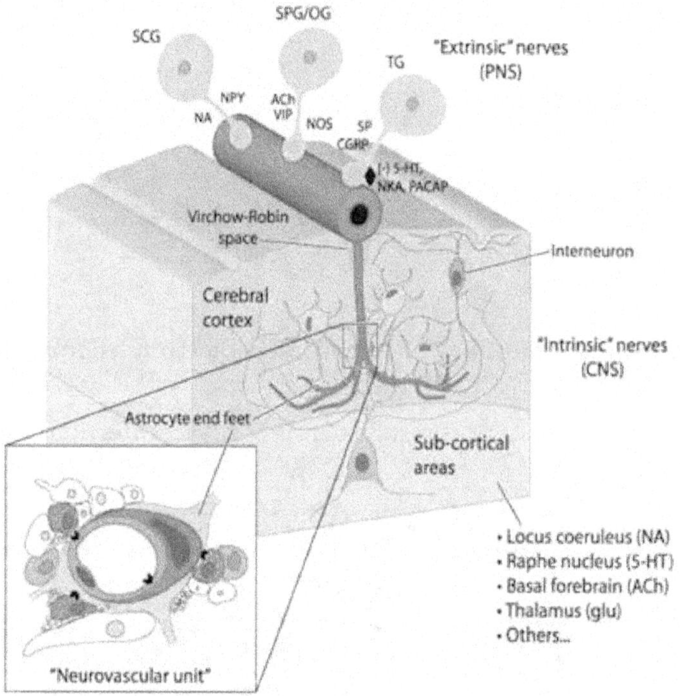

**Figure twenty-four: Brain Injury Complication as a Result of COVID Brain Invasion**

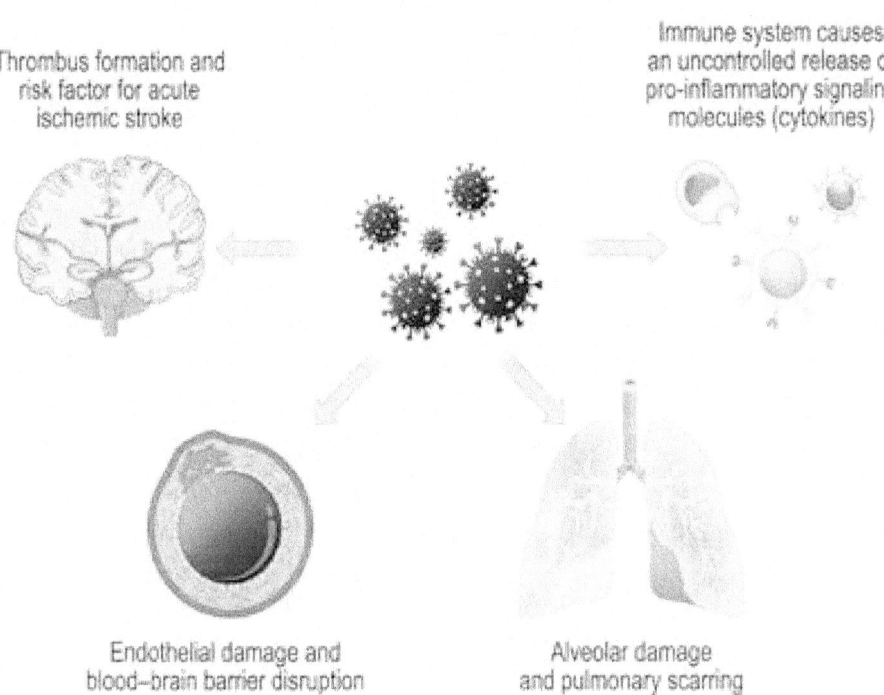

**5**

---

# COVID-19 AND NEUROLOGICAL DISORDER PROBLEMS

**Note:** All listed neurological disorders in the book can be caused by other neurological diseases or existing conditions beside the side effect of COVID-19's previous infection; therefore, patients' physi- cian recommendation and advise is required for additional screening. Treatment options for the listed condition are beyond the scope of this book.

**5.0 Brain Virus Entry Point**

As discussed in section four, SARS-COVID-19 viruses can invade the brain via different paths as the researcher identified:

A- Via Olfactory Path

B- Via blood stream coming from the lung's capillary

C- Brain Blood Barriers

D- COVID-19 virus detected in the CSF

Once the virus enters the brain, it causes damage to the brain cells and triggers neurological disorders as a result. Also, brain cells damaged can be related to the cytosine immune system storms to fight the infection and damages healthy cells around it and cause neurological disorders.

## 5.1 Neurological Disorders Symptoms and Causes

**Table three: Post-COVID-19 Neurological Disorder Some Symptoms Still Under Investigation if COVID Related, this Book will address each Symptom.**

| |
| --- |
| Forgetting about tasks started but did not get completed |
| Taking much longer than usual to complete simple task |
| Feeling frequently distracted |
| Feeling tired when working |
| Needing more time to complete small different tasks |
| Finding Difficulty Sleeping |
| Being more irritable than usual |
| Being frustrated by tasks |
| Anxiety Often Driven by Many Factors Other than Post COVID Infection |
| Forgetting to do things often |
| Headache and being uncommunicative |
| Working on automatic: not thinking |

**Table four: Complete List of Neurological Disorders**

**Note:** Patients can experience one or many symptoms, as listed in **table four**
Some of These Symptoms are still under investigation if COVID related
Patient Physician advised is required

| SID | Post COVID 19 List of Neurological Disorders to Discuss |
|---|---|
| 1 | Forgetting about Task started but did not get Completed Caused By |
| 2 | Taking much longer than usual to complete simple tasks |
| 3 | Feeling frequently distracted |
| 4 | Feeling tired when working |
| 5 | Needing more time to complete small task |
| 6 | Finding Difficulty Sleeping |
| 7 | Being more irritable than usual |
| 8 | Being frustrated by tasks |
| 9 | Anxiety |
| 10 | Depression |
| 11 | Forgetting to do things often |
| 12 | Headache |
| 13 | Being uncommunicative |
| 14 | Working on Automatic not Thinking |
| 15 | Doing tasks in the wrong order |
| 16 | Having difficulty concentrating |

**5.2 Some examples of things a person might do because of brain fog include**

- Forgetting about a task they had to complete
- Taking much longer than usual to complete simple tasks
- Feeling frequently distracted
- Feeling tired when working
- Felling spacey or confused

- Needing more time to complete small tasks

## 5.3 Most Common Brain Fog Symptoms

### Case Study A

- Forgetting about a task they had to complete
- Taking much longer than usual to complete simple tasks
- Feeling frequently distracted
- Feeling tired when working
- Felling spacey or confused
- Needing more time to complete small tasks
- Having difficulty concentrating

## 5.4 Least Common Brain Symptoms

Few reporting available, will not be addressed for insufficient data

### Case Study B

- Doing tasks in the wrong order
- Finding difficulty to do multi tasks at the same time
- Forgetting to do things often
- Working on automatic; not thinking
- Headache
- Memory Concentration
- Depression or anxiety
- Feeling tired or yawning all the time
- Being more irritable than usual
- Being frustrated by tasks

# Figure twenty-five: Long Term Effects of COVID-19

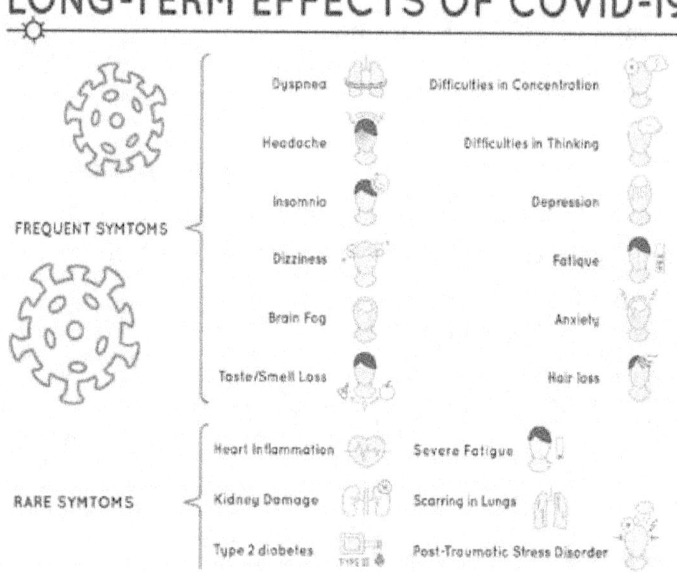


## 5.5 Brain Lobes Function as Related to Brain Fog Symptoms

## Table six: Brain Parts Functional Description

| Frontal lobe | Parietal lobe |
| --- | --- |
| Personality, behavior, emotions | Interprets language, words |
| Judgment, planning, problem solving | Sense of touch, pain, temperature |
| Speech: speaking and writing (Broca's area) | Interprets signals from vision, hearing, and memory |
| Body movement (motor strip) | **Temporal lobe** |
| Intelligence, concentration, self-awareness | Understanding language |
| **Occipital lobe** | Memory |
| Interprets vision (color, light, movement) | Hearing |
| | Sequencing and organization |

BRAIN FUNCTION
INFOGRAPHIC
FRONTAL LOBE
intelligence
problem solving
reading
speaking
language
sensation
body orientation
reading
sensation
knowing right and left
PARIENTAL LOBE
OCCIPITAL LOBE
vision
color perception
TEMPORAL LOBE
behaviour
intelligence
memory
movement
hearing
CEREBELLUM
ballance
coordination
muscle control
SPINAL CORD
breathing
body temperature
digestion
swallowing
sleep

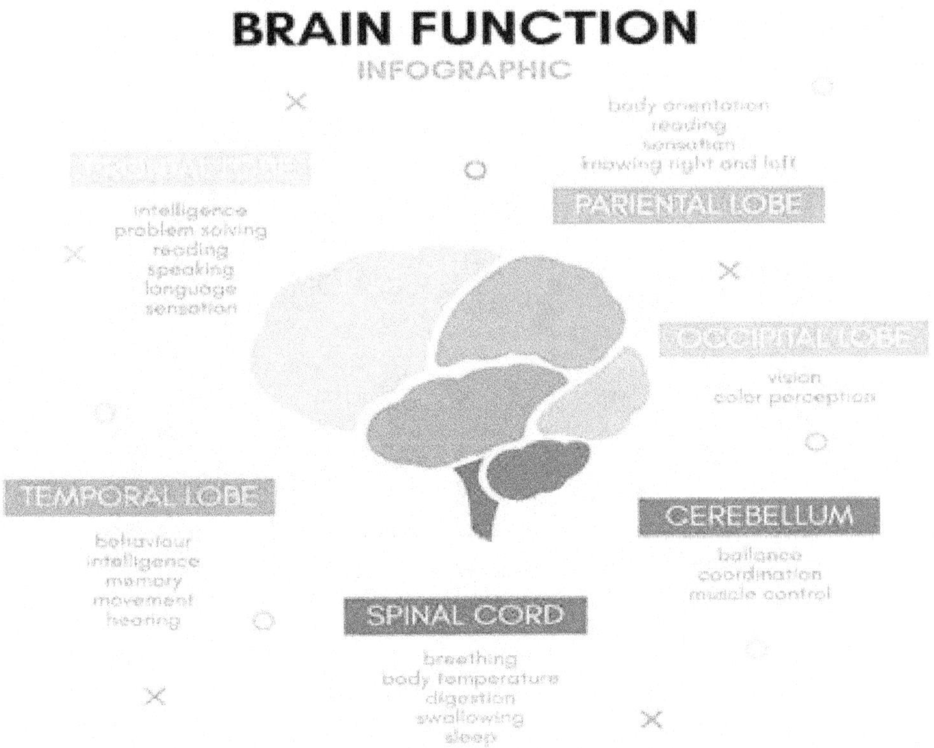

**Figure twenty-seven: Amygdala in the brain, and close-up view of amygdala neurons, 3D illustration.**

Two almond- shaped clusters of nuclei within temporal lobes, part of the limbic system, play a role in memory and emotions.

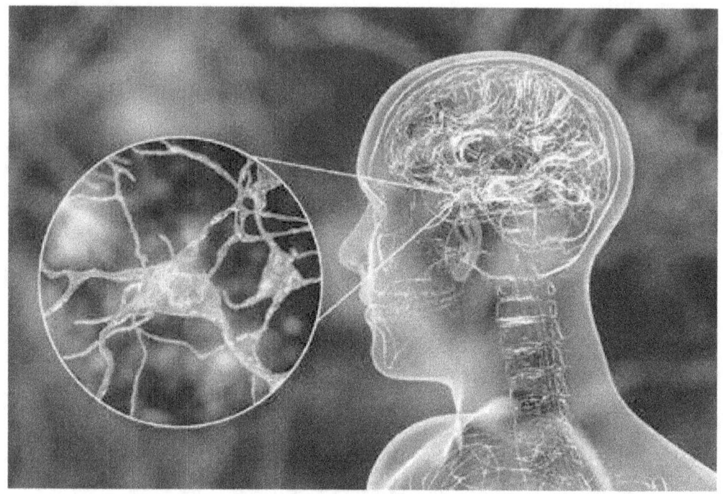

**Figure twenty-eight:** Brain Lobes Location

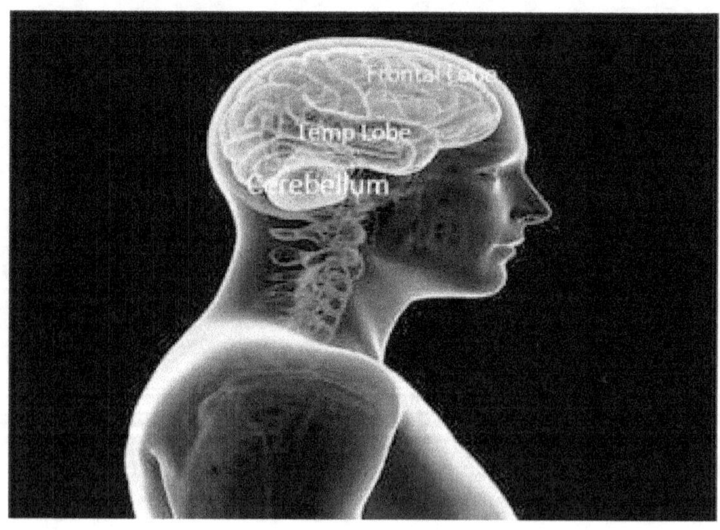

Figure twenty-nine: Frontal Lobe Visualized Location

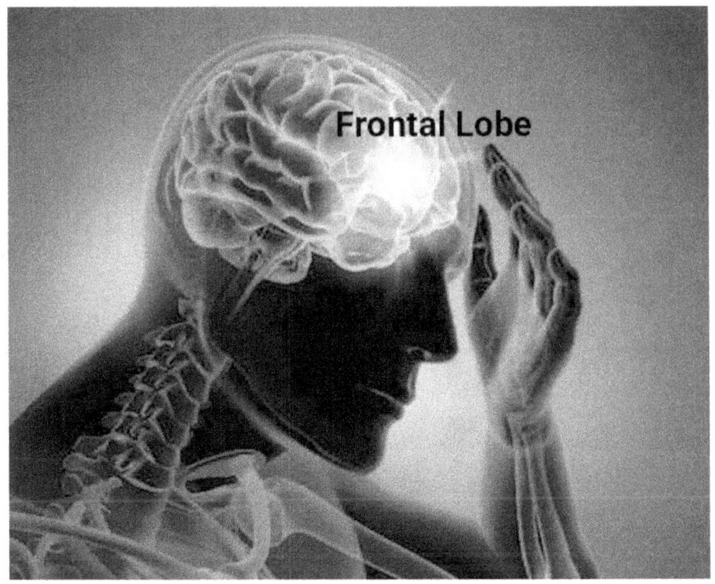



Figure thirty: Brain Right and Left Functional Description

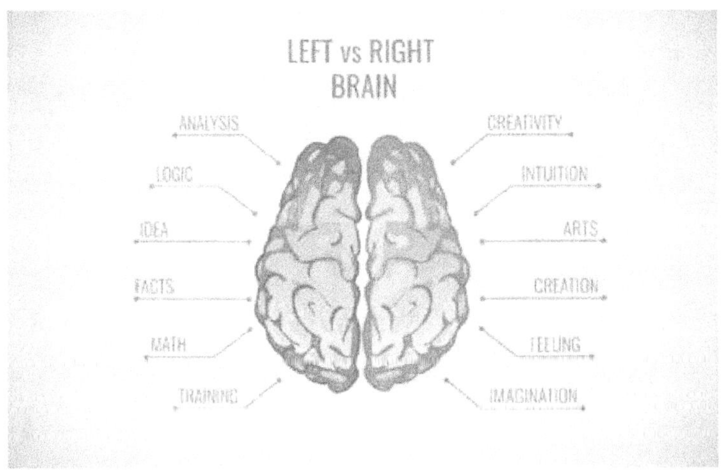

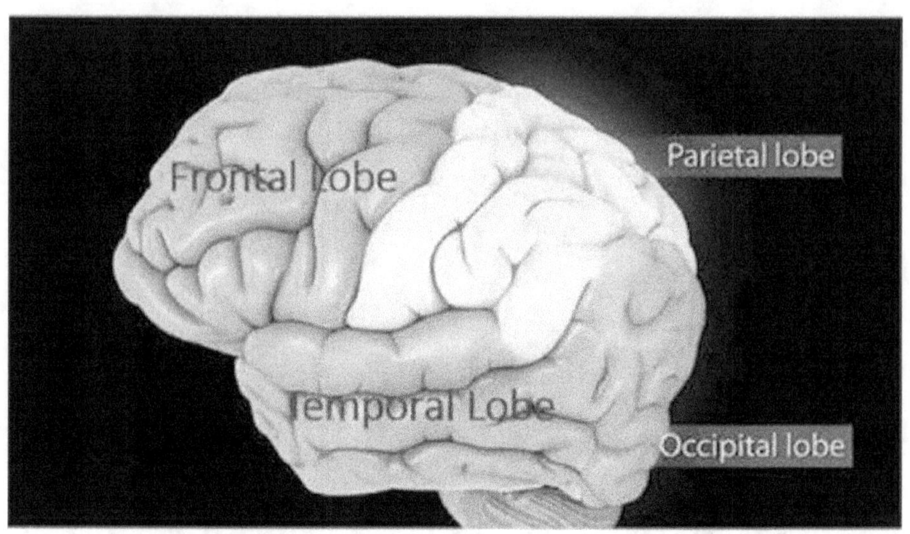

Frontal Lobe
Parietal lobe
Temporal Lobe
Occipital lobe

**6**

---

# POST COVID-19 BRAIN FOG DIAGNOSIS

**6.0 This section will address the most common brain fog symptoms following past COVID infection**

**Table seven: Brain Fog Most Common Symptoms.**

**Note:** All listed symptoms below are still under further investigation and clinical research.

- Forgetting about a task they had to complete
- Taking much longer than usual to complete simple tasks
- Feeling frequently distracted
- Feeling tired when working
- Felling spacey or confused
- Needing more time to complete small tasks
- Having difficulty concentrating

## 6.1 Brain Fog: What causes it?

Brain Fog is the first item to discuss as a result of post-COVID infections.

In some patients, COVID can cause brain injury, such as stroke, and you would have persistent deficits or problems related to that stroke. But some people seem to have this brain fog out of proportion to their illness. They had a mild illness and they recovered, except they continue to have long-lasting cognitive problems. A study

suspected this could be due to immune system activation, such that the immune system releases these molecules that help to make the immune system function and fight infections, but as a side effect, the immune system attack can impact the nervous system, **damages Glial cells and Astrocytes,** which results in interrupting the neuron communication to perform its tasks.

### 6.1.1 Brain Fog Causes Rather than post-COVID-19 Infection

Several factors and health conditions can cause brain fog, not related to post-COVID infection, including:

- Lack of sleep
- Increased stress levels
- Depression
- Dementia
- Perimenopause
- Medication side effects such as painkillers and others; doc- tors should evaluate patient medications and their side effects
- Hormonal conditions, such as thyroid disorders
- Chronic health conditions, such as multiple sclerosis
- Nutrient deficiencies, such as a vitamin $B_{12}$ deficiency

**7**

---

# SYMPTOM ONE

## FORGETTING ABOUT TASKS STARTED BUT NOT COMPLETED

Identifying the brain's damaged parts can relate to symptom one.

A physician should evaluate the patient by going through the process listed below:

A- Short-term memory damages evaluation

B- Prefrontal lobe damage evaluation

C- Astrocyte's damage evaluation

D- Microglia damage by SARS-CoV-2 infection

E-Glia cells damage control MRI screening

F-Performing Enhanced MRI Scanning for above listed items

*The List of Brain Parts that Can Cause Symptom One: memory, Prefrontal lobe, and Astrocytes*

## 7.1 Brain short-term memory damages evaluation

Brain short-term memory damages evaluation, also called working memory, and occurs in the prefrontal cortex. It stores information for about one minute, and its capacity is limited to about seven items. For example, doctor should ask patient if he or she can dial a phone number someone just told him from a list of seven items.

## 7.2 Concentration Prefrontal Lobe Damage

The front of the brain behind the forehead is the frontal lobe. The frontal lobe is the part of the brain that helps people to organize, plan, pay attention, focus, and make decisions.

Astrocytes damage evaluation and are master regulators of synaptic activity. Astrocyte-neuron signaling, which supports the wide range of functional consequences of astrocytes on synaptic transmission and behavior. Current data show that astrocytes, via expression of ion channels, neurotransmitter receptors, subcellular Ca2+.

## 7.3 Astrocytes

Neurons talk to each other across synapses. When an action potential reaches the presynaptic terminal, it causes neurotransmitters to be released from the neuron into the synaptic cleft, a 20–40 nm gap between the presynaptic axon terminal and the postsynaptic dendrite (often a spine) needed for communicating between two neurons.

## 7.4 Microglia

Microglia damage SARS-CoV-2 infection or COVID-19. Within the central nervous system (CNS), microglia act as the central housekeepers against altered homeostatic states, including during viral neurotropic infections. In this review, we highlight microglial responses to viral neuro infections, especially those with a similar genetic composition and route of entry as SARS-CoV-2. As the primary sensor of viral infection in the CNS, we describe these as pathogenic and microinvasive.

## 7.5 Glia damage control

Evaluation of the formation of synaptic circuits in the CNS: glial cells are in tight association with synapses in all brain regions. Astrocytes and microglia are ramified cells that extend numerous small processes that associate with synapses. Glial processes are proposed to actively participate in the regulation of synaptic transmission.

**Figure thirty-one: Neurological Cells Anatomy Illustration**

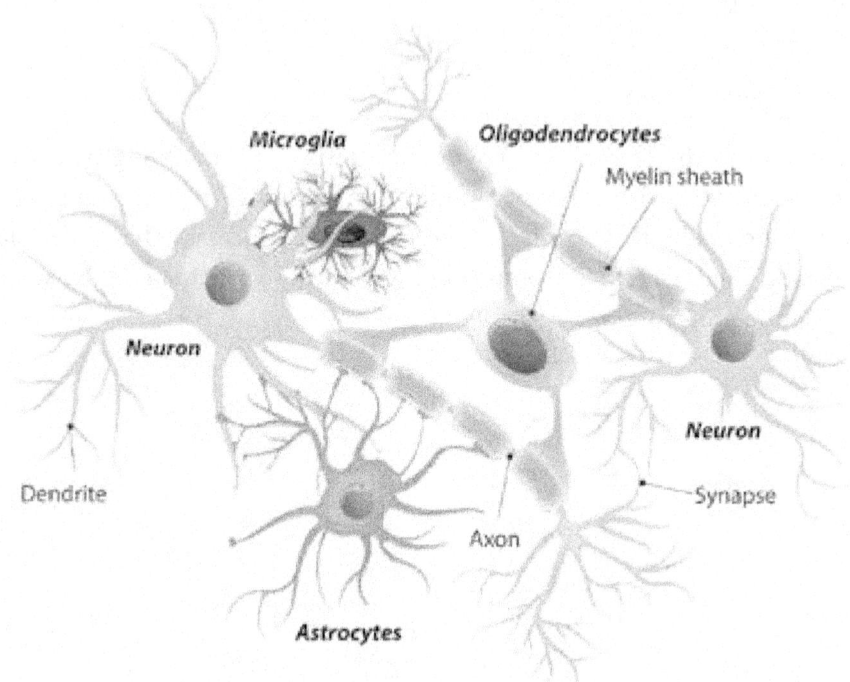


## 7.6 Imaging Diagnosis for Symptom One

In this section we will address the first symptoms of brain fog which is forgetting about task started but did not get completed. Symptom's diagnosis will include advance MRI imaging of brain frontal and temporal lobe for any cell's damages.

# Figure thirty-two: Glia Cells Damages under Electron Microscope

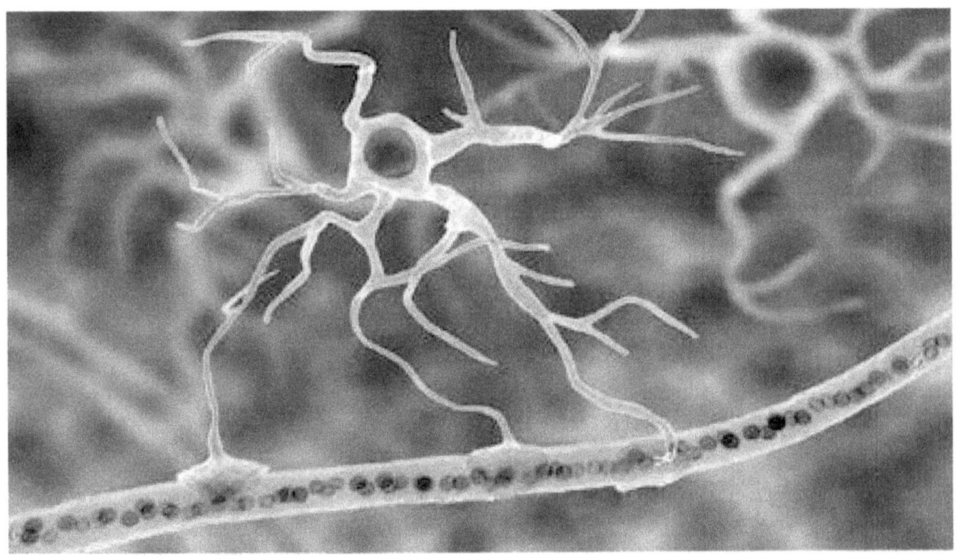

# Figure thirty-three: Brain Cells Astrocytes and Neuron Interrelationship Anatomy Illustration

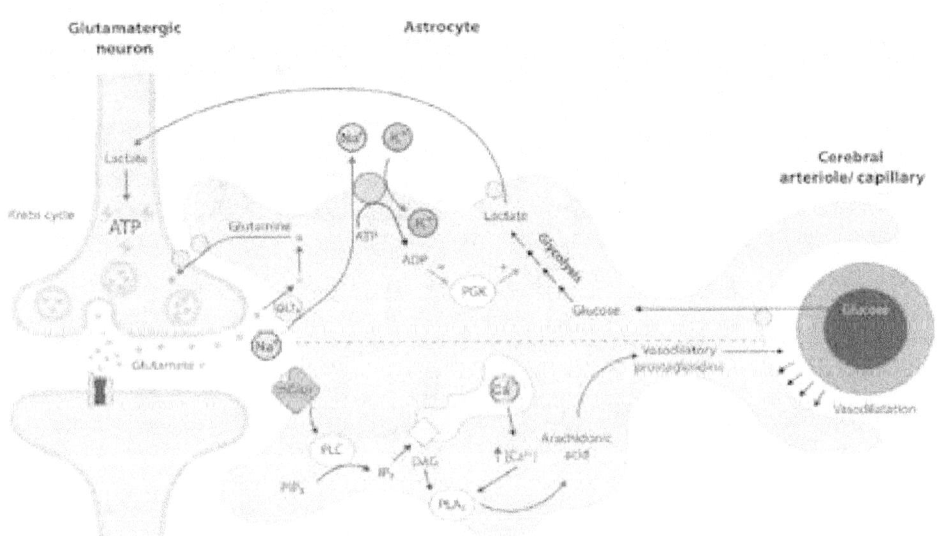

### 7.7.1 MRI Advance Imaging Diagnose for Brain Fog Symptom One

Symptom One Diagnosis and Enhanced MRI Sample Imaging

**Figure thirty-four: Ischemic stroke followed severe COVID infection.**

CT of the brain showed cerebral infarction at left frontal, temporal, parietal lobe at cross-sectional imaging.

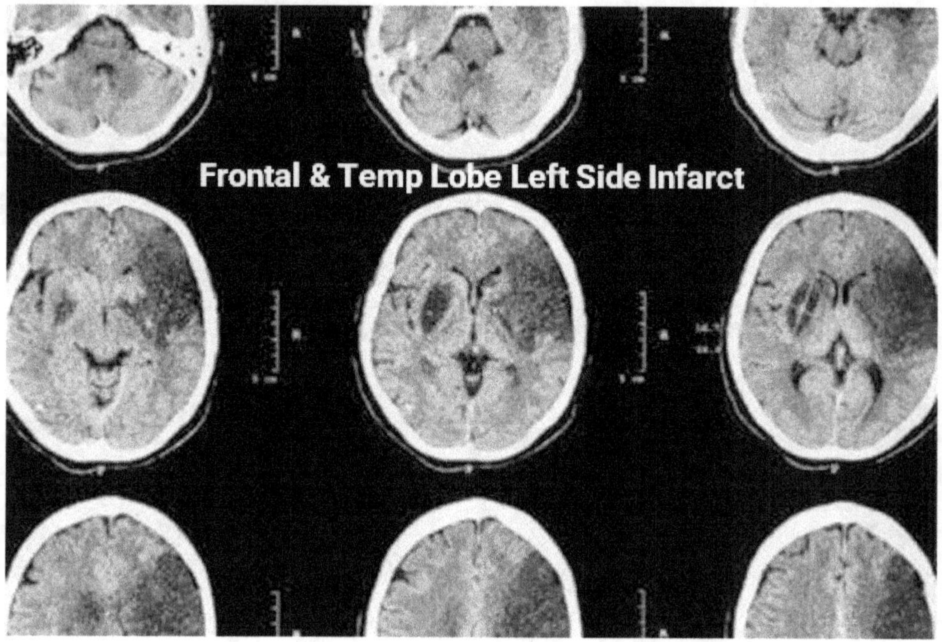

# Figure thirty-five: Multi MRI Scan for Frontal and Temp Lobes Infarct

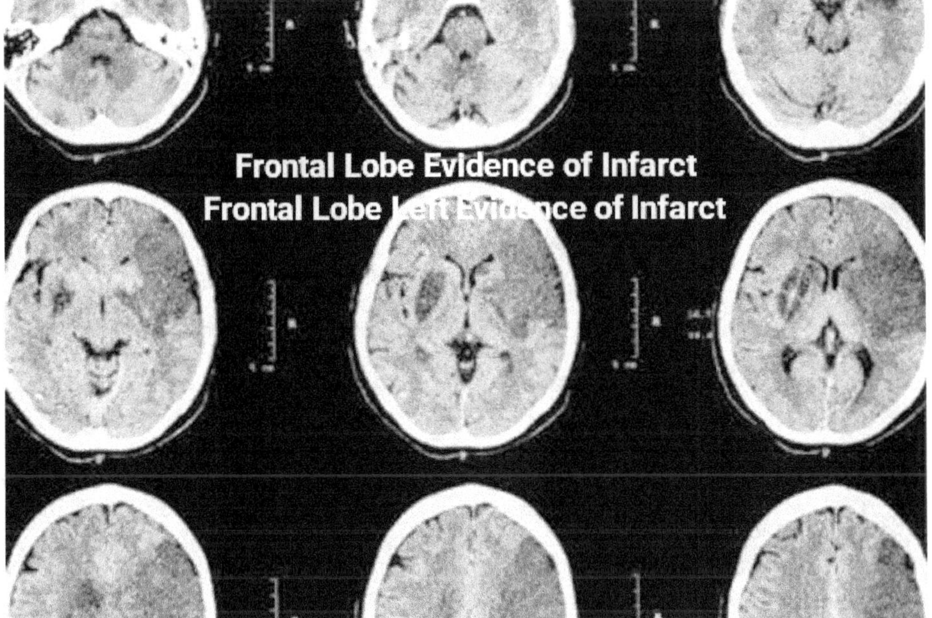

# Figure thirty-six: Multi MRI Scan for Frontal and Temp Lobes Infarct (Sample Image)

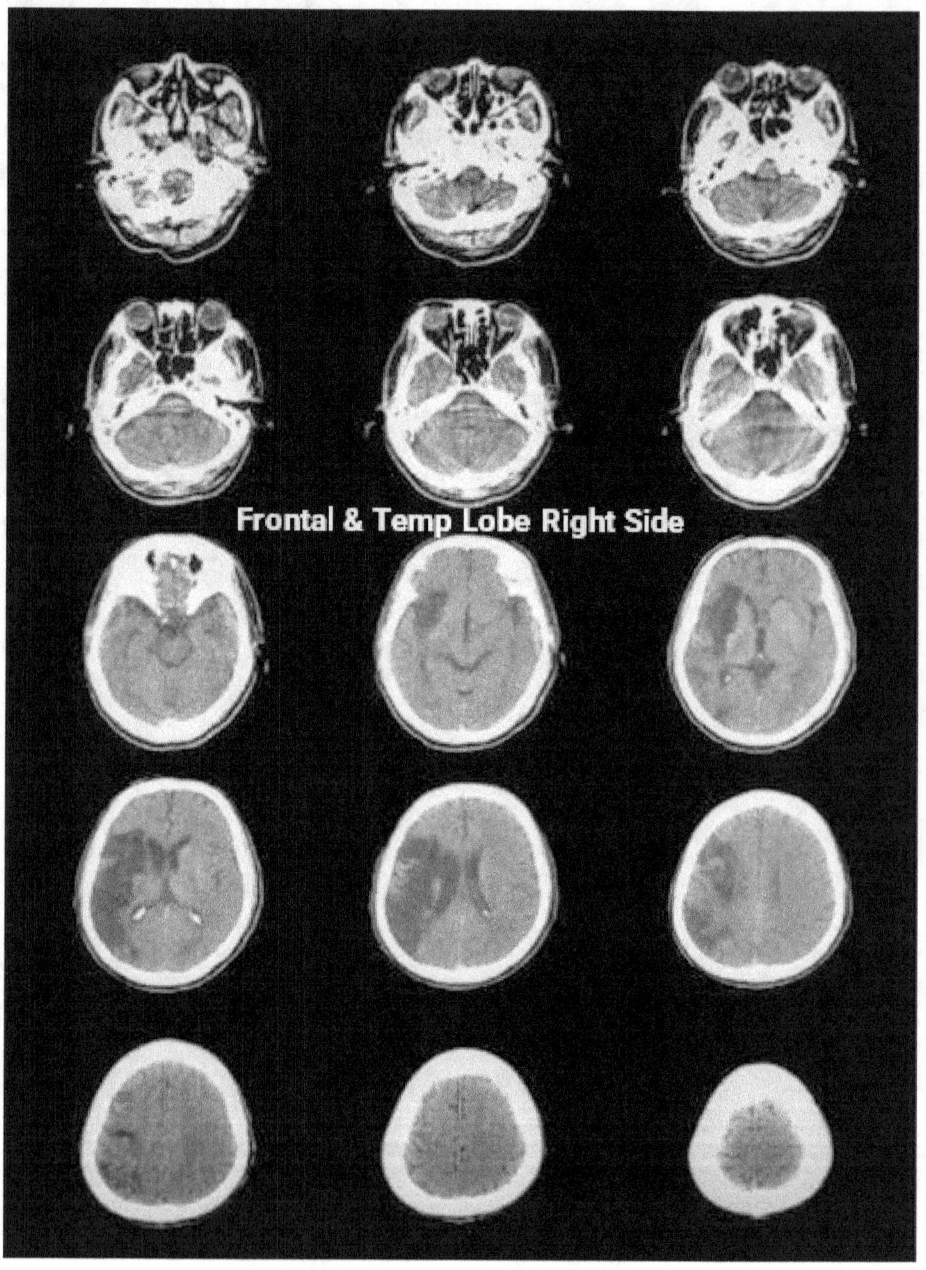

**8**

---

# SYMPTOM TWO

## TAKING MUCH LONGER THAN USUAL TO COMPLETE SIMPLE TASKS

**Identifying brain-damaged parts can relate to symptom two**

**8.0 This symptom can be related to different factors rather than post-COVID infections as:**

Whether you've had enough sleep, if you've had less than six hours, it's harder for your *brain* to tune out distractions and focus long enough to finish what you need to do.

Other signs that you need more shutting eyes include:

- Falling asleep while watching TV or reading a book
- Feeling irritable
- Sleeping longer on weekends
- Trouble waking up in the mornings

**List of Brain Parts Can Cause Symptom Two:** lateral prefrontal cortex, PFC

What part of the brain is responsible for performing tasks and can be infected by COVID virus?

- **The rostro lateral prefrontal cortex (RLPFC)** is an area of neurons that sits in the front of the brain.
- **Prefrontal Cortex,** the Prefrontal Cortex (PFC) and hip- pocampus are the most critical parts of the human brain for decision making, which are the parts of the brain allow ing you to multitask.

**Symptom Two Diagnosis and Enhanced MRI Imaging**

**8.1 Physician Performs Imaging Diagnosis for Symptom two as Related to Post-COVID Infection**

**Figure thirty-seven: Evidence of PFC Degradation Enhanced MRI Sample Imaging**

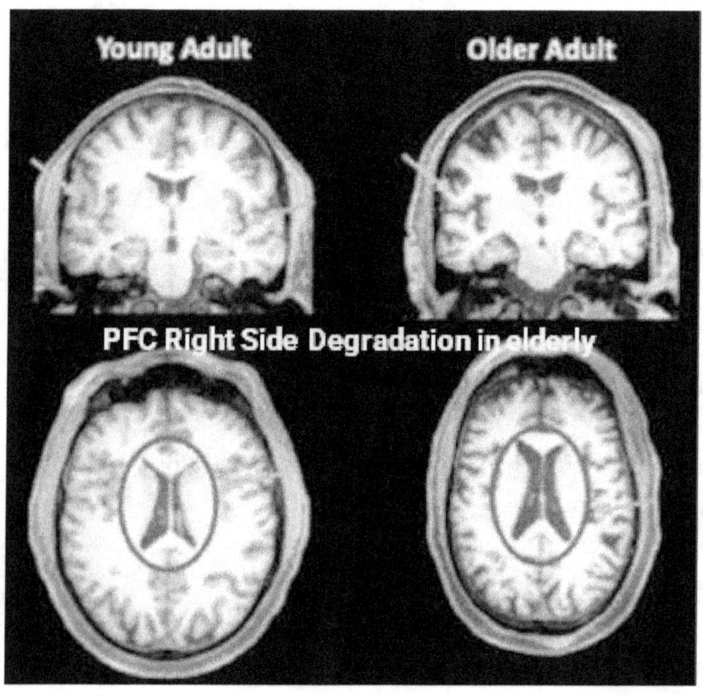

9

———————

# SYMPTOM THREE
## FEELING FREQUENTLY DISTRACTED

**Identifying brain damaged parts can relate to symptom three.**

**9.1 Experience occasional brain fog and anxiety**

Experience occasional brain fog and anxiety, especially during times of high stress. However, people who find that anxiety and brain fog regularly interfere with their everyday activities, it can be related to POS-COVID infection neurological disorder.

**Figure thirty-eight: Which Parts of the Brain Responsible for Concentration**

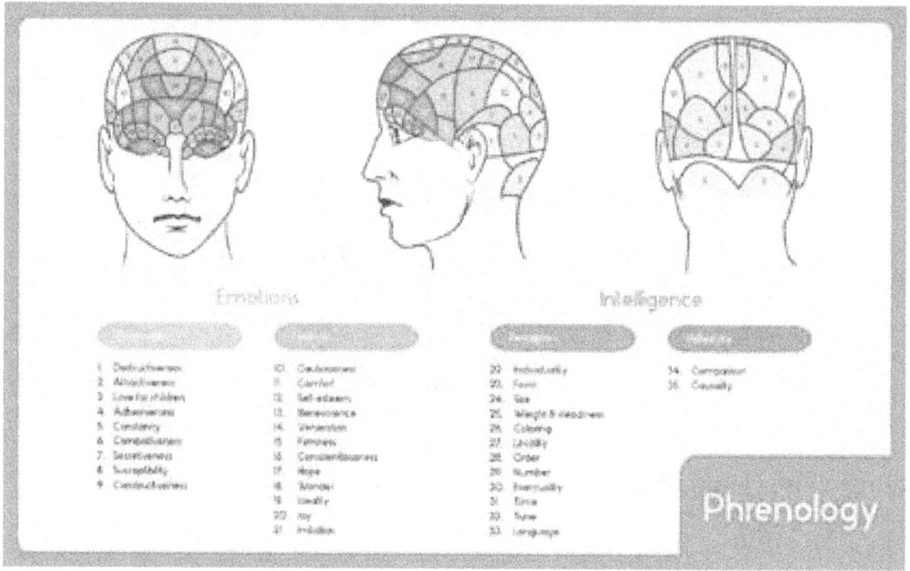



**Symptom Three Diagnosis and Enhanced MRI Imaging**

**List of Brain Parts that Can Cause Symptom Three: Prefrontal cortex**

**9.2 Physician Performs Enhanced MRI Imaging**

Physician Performs Enhanced MRI Imaging for prefrontal cortex for any inflammation as a result of post-COVID infection.

Figure thirty-nine: MRI Scan for Prefrontal Cortex Evidence of Inflammation

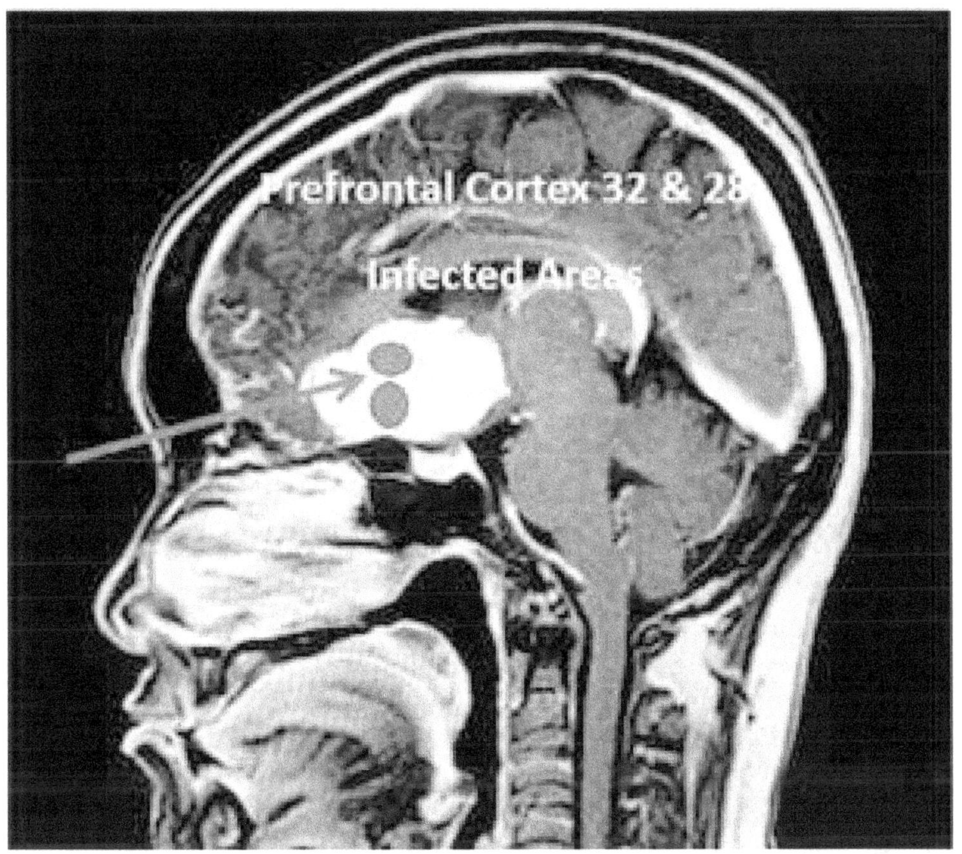

**10**

---

# SYMPTOM FOUR

## FEELING TIRED WHEN WORKING

**Identifying brain damaged parts can relate to symptom four.**

**10.1 Coronavirus potentially triggering chronic fatigue syndrome**

A significant proportion of COVID-19 patients are suffering from prolonged post-COVID-19 Fatigue Syndrome, with characteristics typically found in Myalgic Encephalomyelitis / Chronic Fatigue Syndrome (ME/CFS). However, no clear pathophysiological explanation has yet been provided. For a post-COVID-19 Fatigue Syndrome, which could be targeting a *stress-integrator* within the brain: the hypothalamic, it is proposed that inflammatory mediators released at the site of COVID-19 infection would be transmitted as *stress-signals* in genetically susceptible people.

**List of Brain Parts Can Cause Symptom Four: Hypothalamus**

**Figure forty: Hypothalamus Stress Response Anatomy Illustration**

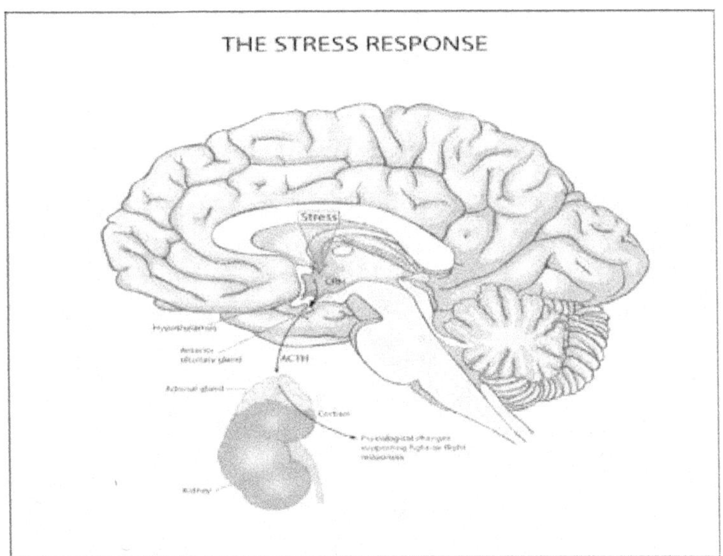


**Symptom Four Diagnosis and Enhanced MRI Imaging**

## 10.2 Physician Performs Enhanced MRI Imaging for Hypothalamus as a Result of Stress Syndrome

**Figure forty-one: Diagnosis for Hypothalamus MRI Scan evidence of any previous damaged as a result of post-COVID infection**

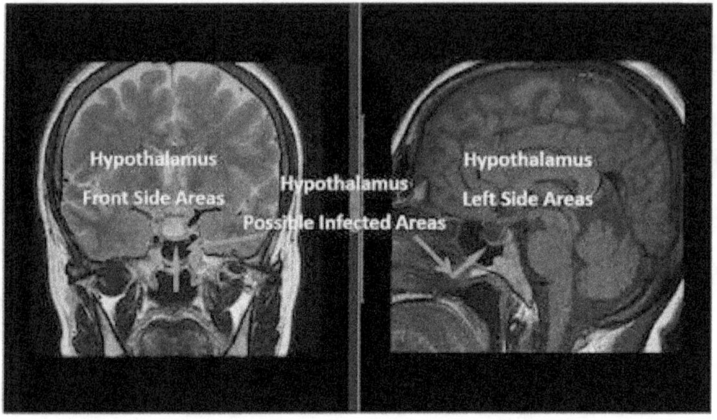

**11**

---

# SYMPTOM FIVE

## NEEDING MORE TIME TO COMPLETE SMALL TASKS

**Identifying brain damaged parts can relate to symptom five.**

**11.1 Attention-deficit hyperactivity disorder affects behavior**

People who have it often have trouble making decisions or getting tasks done before a deadline. Some get too distracted by other activities around them. Others find it hard to plan, or they get frustrated easily and give up.

Based on previous research showing widespread changes in the brain macro and microstructure, it was hypothesized that an adult ADHD diagnosis is associated with **frontal, basal ganglia, anterior** cingu- late, **temporal, and parietal regions** in COVID-19 patients.

**ADHD** is associated with abnormally low levels of the

neurotransmitters transmitting between the prefrontal cortical area and the **basal ganglia.**

**List of Brain Parts Can Cause Symptom Five:** Anterior cingulate, Frontal, basal ganglia, cingulate temporal and parietal Region

## 11.2 Brain Areas to be Examined

- Anterior cingulate
- Frontal, basal ganglia
- Temporal and parietal regions

**Figure forty-two: Anterior cingulate Anatomy Illustration**

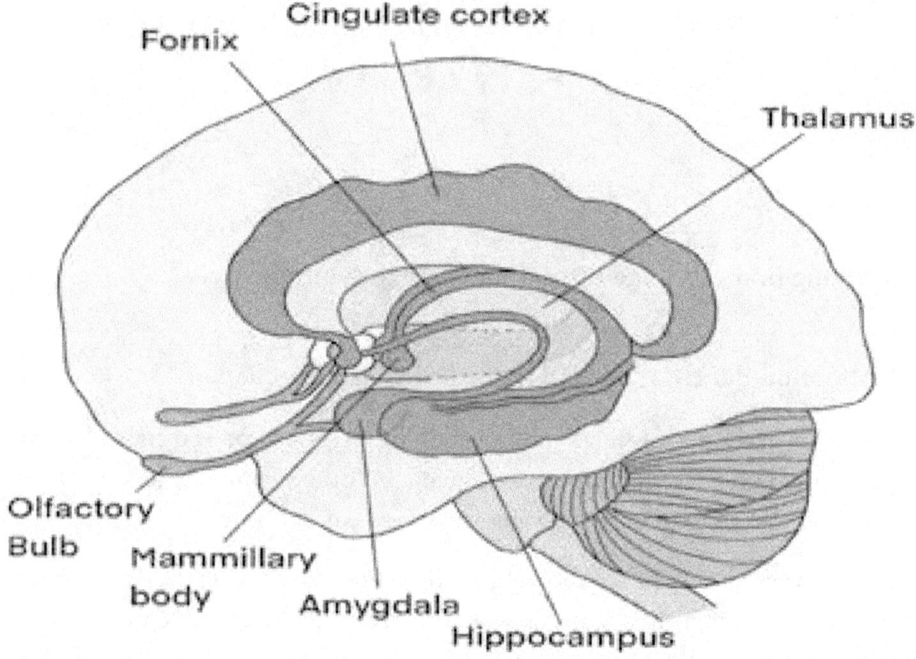

## 11.3 Frontal, basal ganglia Anatomy Illustration

MRI: Brain shows right sphenoid ridge meningioma with mass effect to right frontal lobe, right basal ganglia, and triliteral ventricle.

**Figure forty-three: Front Ganglia AnatomySymptom Five Diagnosis and Enhance MRI Imaging**

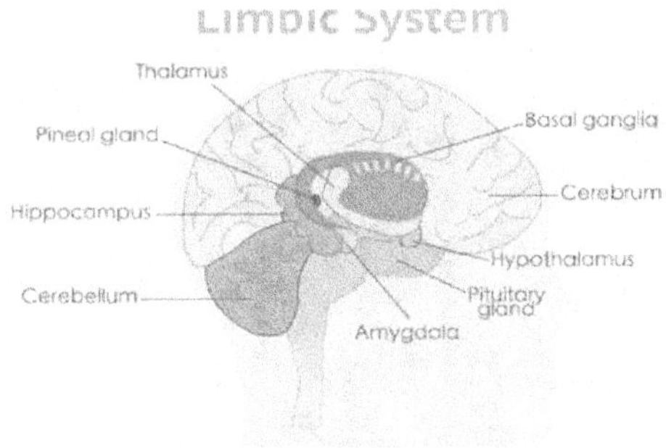


Limbic system

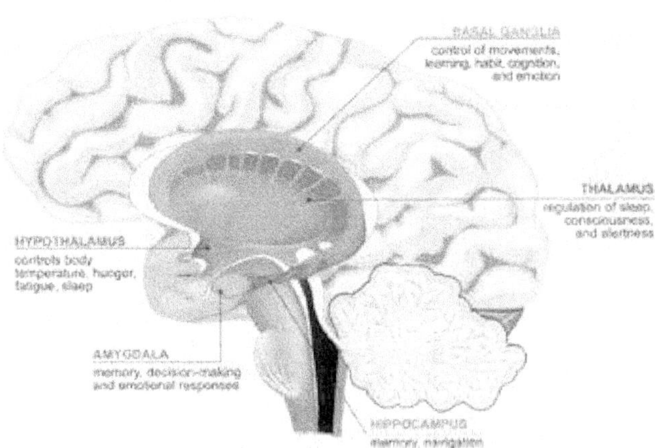

## 11.4 Physician Performs Enhanced MRI Scan for Ganglia

To locate any evidence of inflammation or damages caused by previous COVID infection.

**Figure forty-four: Enhanced MRI Sample scan of Basal Ganglia Evidence of Post-COVID Infection**

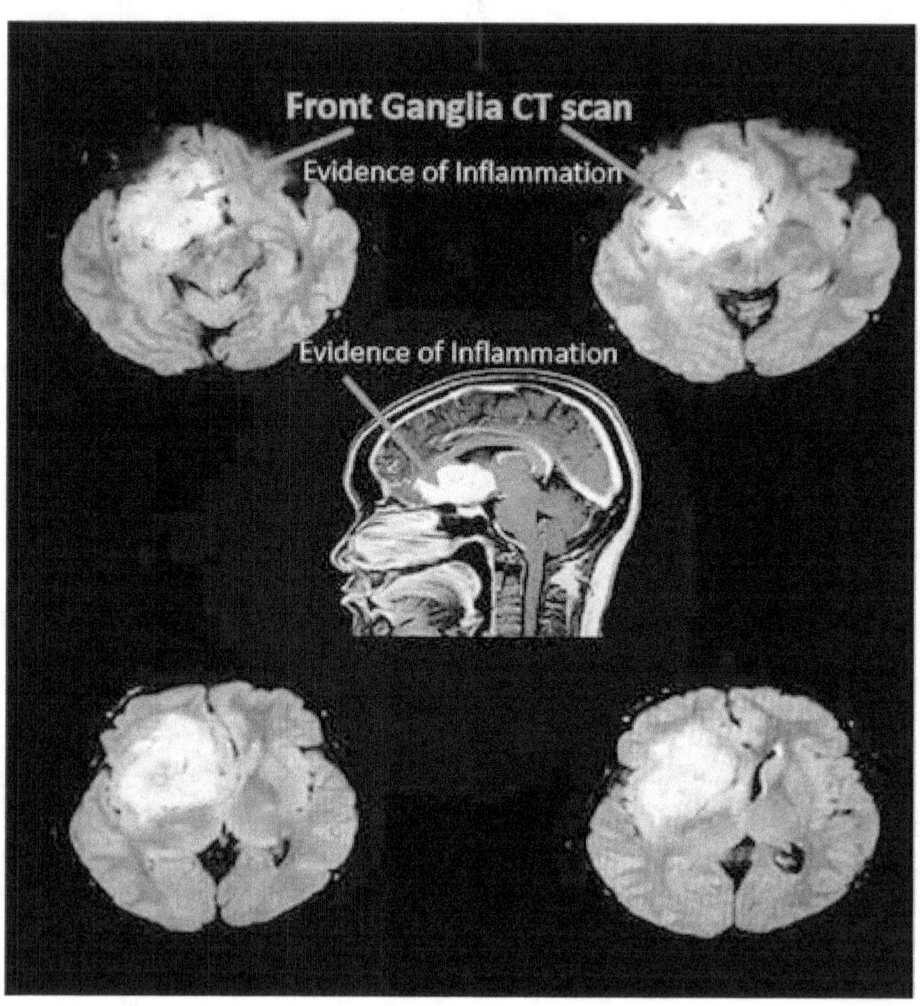

**12**

---

# SYMPTOM SIX

## FINDING DIFFICULTY SLEEPING

**Identifying brain damaged parts can relate to symptom six.**

**12.1 Difficulties Sleeping due to COVID Infection.**

Many people who have brain injuries suffer from sleep disturbances. **Not sleeping well can increase or worsen depression, anxiety, fatigue, irritability, and one's sense of well-being.** It can also lead to poor work performance and traffic or workplace accidents.

**List of Brain Parts that Can Cause Symptom Six:** Hypothalamus, Thalamus, Pineal Glands

**12.2 Brain Parts Responsible for Sleeping**

The **hypothalamus**, a peanut-sized structure deep inside the brain, contains groups of nerve cells that act as control centers affect- ing sleep and arousal. Within the hypothalamus **suprachiasmatic nucleus** (SCN), clusters of thousands of cells that receive information about light exposure directly from the eyes and control your behavioral rhythm.

The **thalamus.** During most stages of sleep, the thalamus becomes quiet, letting you tune out the external world. But during REM sleep, the thalamus is active, sending the cortex images, sounds, and other sensations that fill our dreams.

The **pineal gland**, located within the brain's two hemispheres, receives signals from the SCN and increases production of the hor- mone *melatonin*, which helps put you to sleep once the lights go down.

The **basal forebrain**, near the front and bottom of the brain, also promotes sleep and wakefulness, while part of the **midbrain** acts as an arousal system.

The **amygdala**, an almond-shaped structure involved in processing emotions, becomes increasingly active during REM sleep.

## 12.3 Brain Parts Involved in Sleeping Anatomy Illustration

**Figure forty-five: Pineal Glands Anatomy**

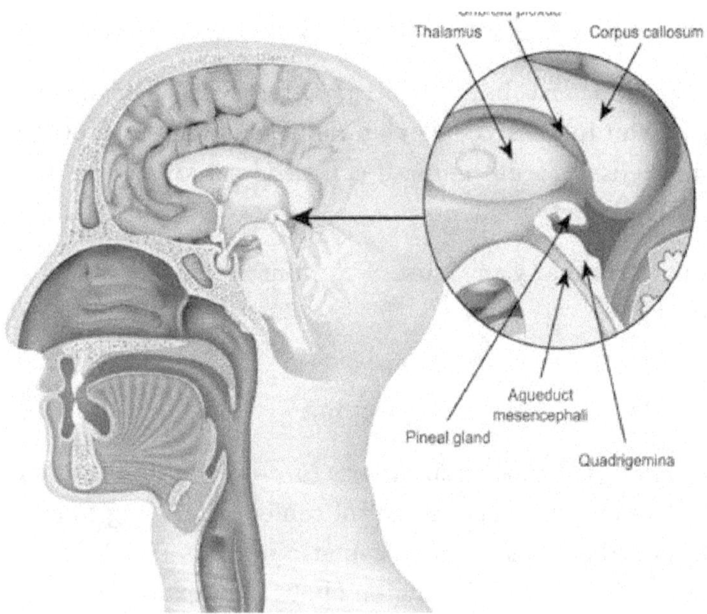

Symptom Six Diagnosis and Enhance MRI Imaging

## 12.4 Sleep Deprivation Caused by Post-COVID Infection

**Figure forty-six: Physician performs enhanced MRI Sample scanning for evidence of any damage to the brain hypothalamus gland as a result of post-COVID infection**

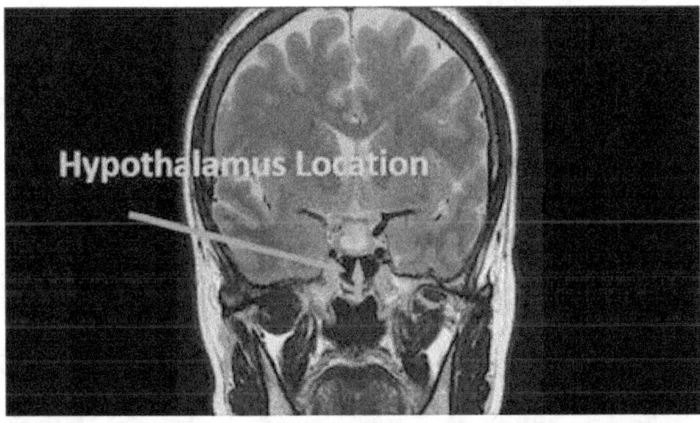


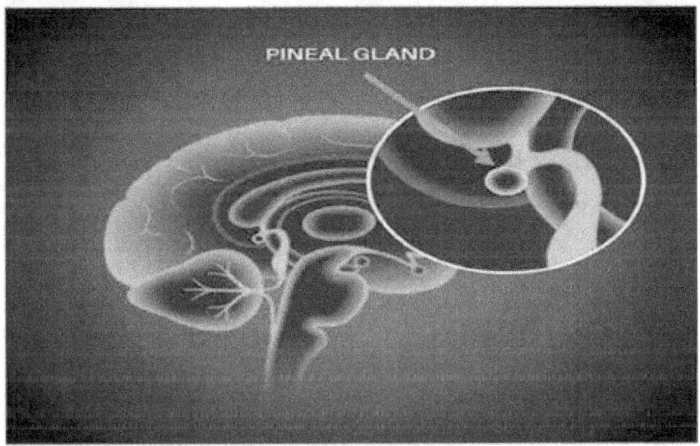

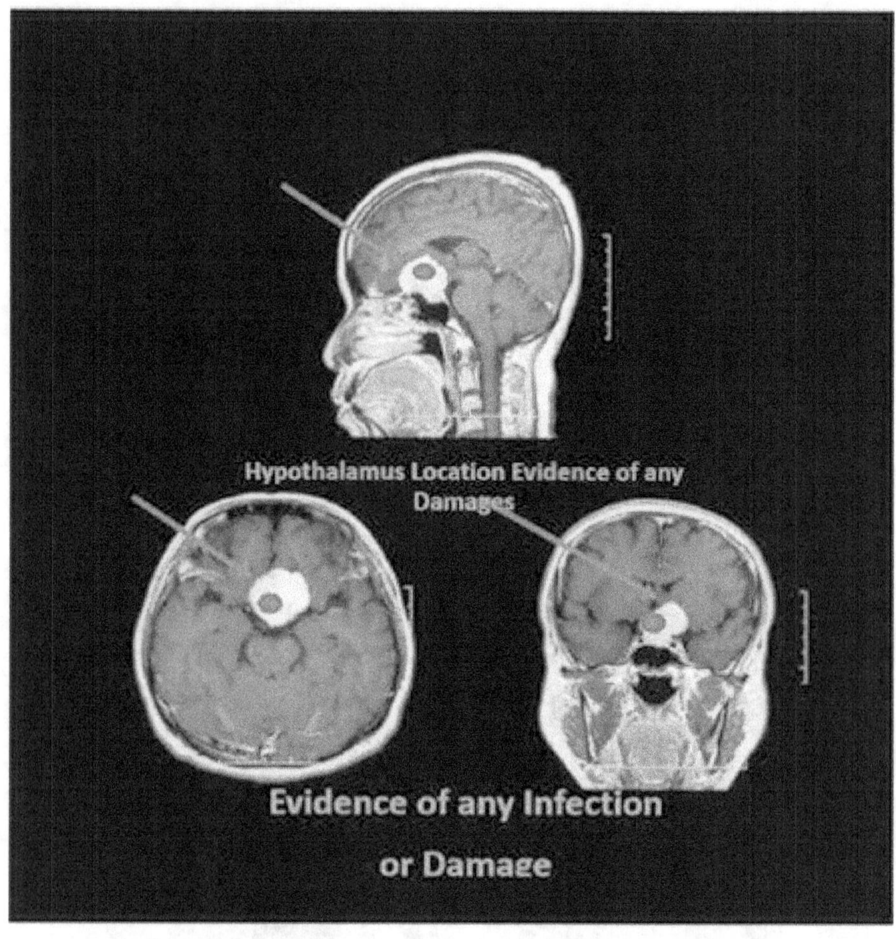


Hypothalamus Location Evidence of any Damages
Evidence of any Infection or Damage

**13**

---

# BEING MORE IRRITABLE THAN USUAL

**Identifying brain damaged parts can relate to symptom seven.**

**13.1 Irritability is a common emotion.**

Many factors can cause or contribute to **irritability**, including life stress, a lack of sleep, or low blood.

The amygdala is **responsible** for processing strong emotions, such as fear, pleasure, or anger. It might also send signals to the **cerebral** cortex.

**A cluster of almond-shaped cells located near the base of the brain.** Everyone has two of these cell groups, one in each hemisphere (or side) of the brain. **The amygdalae help define and regulate emotions.**

**List of Brain Parts Can Cause Symptom Seven:** Amygdala, Limbic System

The amygdala is **a complex structure of cells nestled in the middle of the brain, adjacent to the hippocampus** (which is associated with memory formation). The amygdala is primarily involved in the processing of emotions and memories associated with fear.

## 13.2 Damaged Amygdala as a result of post-COVID Infection, MRI Scan

**Figure forty-eight: Amygdala Location**

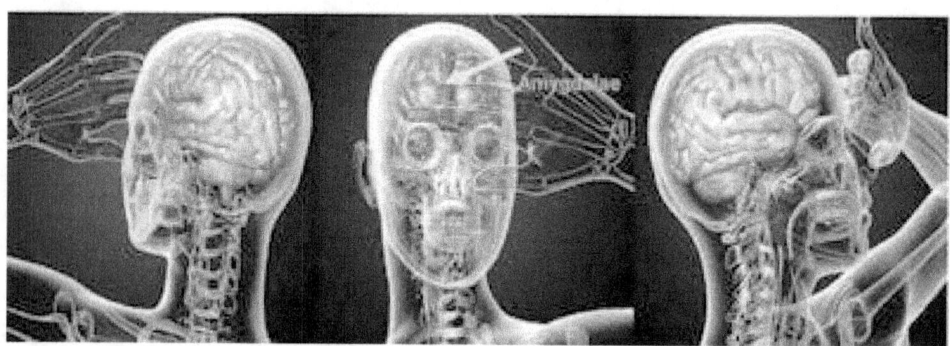

**Figure forty-nine: Limbic System Glands Details Anatomy Illustration**

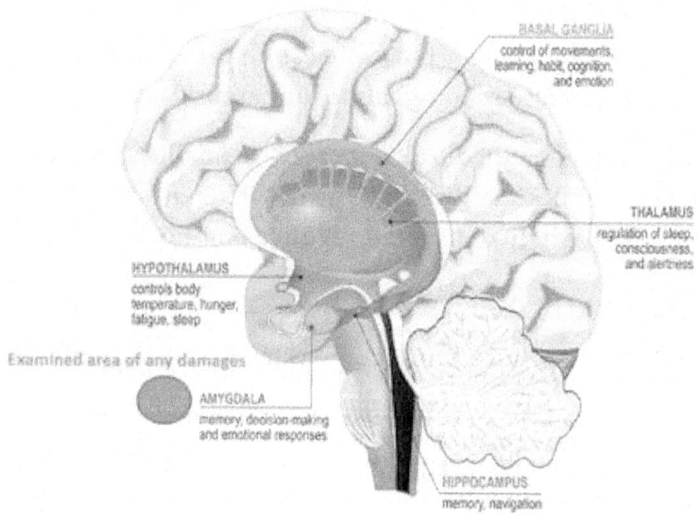

# Figure fifty: Enhanced MRI Amygdala Sample Scan

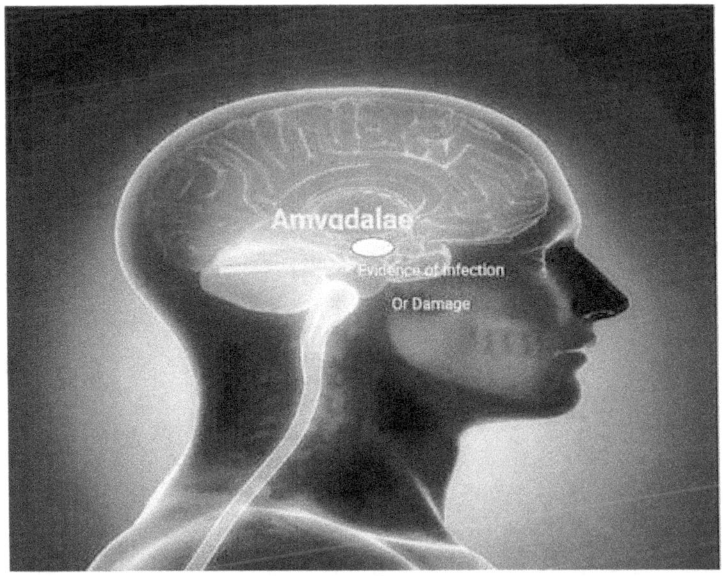


# Figure fifty-one: cerebral cortex (Sample Scan)

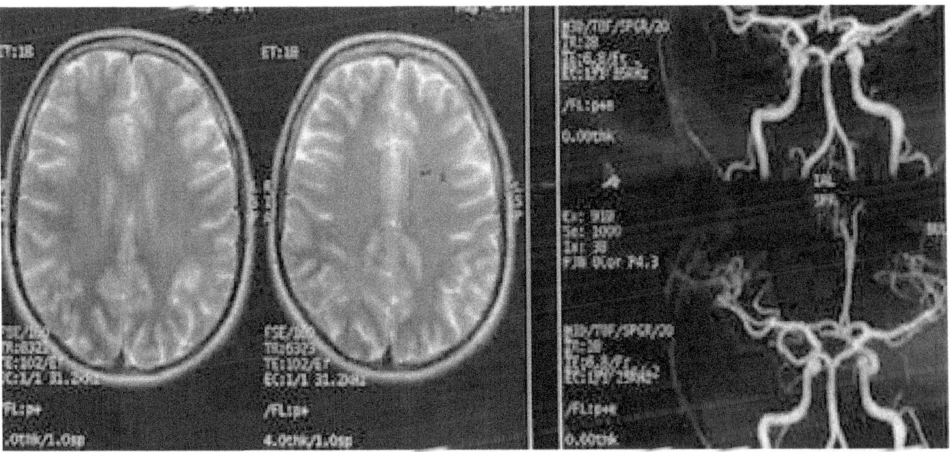

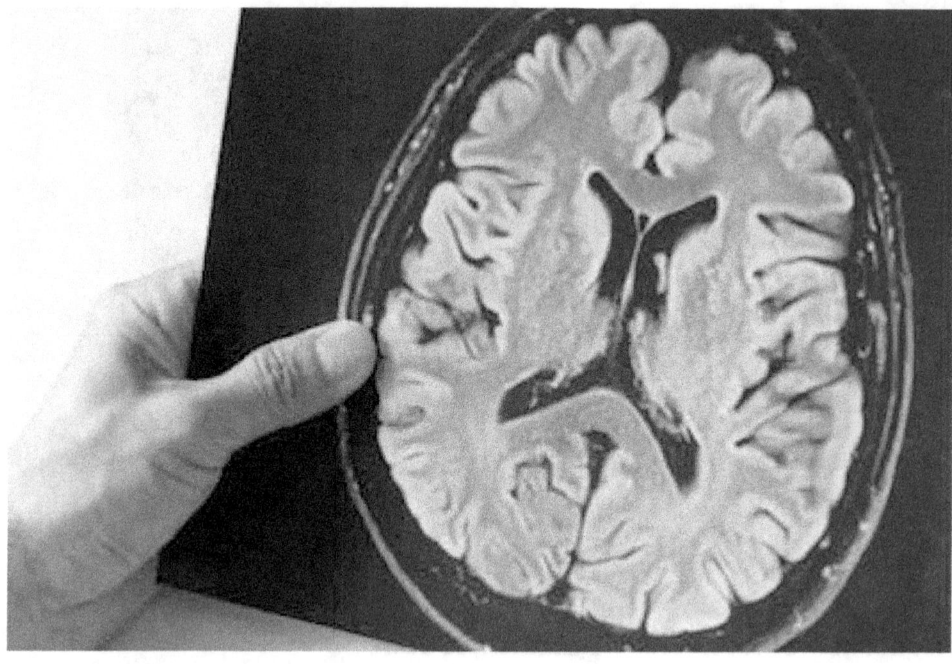

**Cerebral Cortex Blood Clots as Result from COVID Severe Infection**

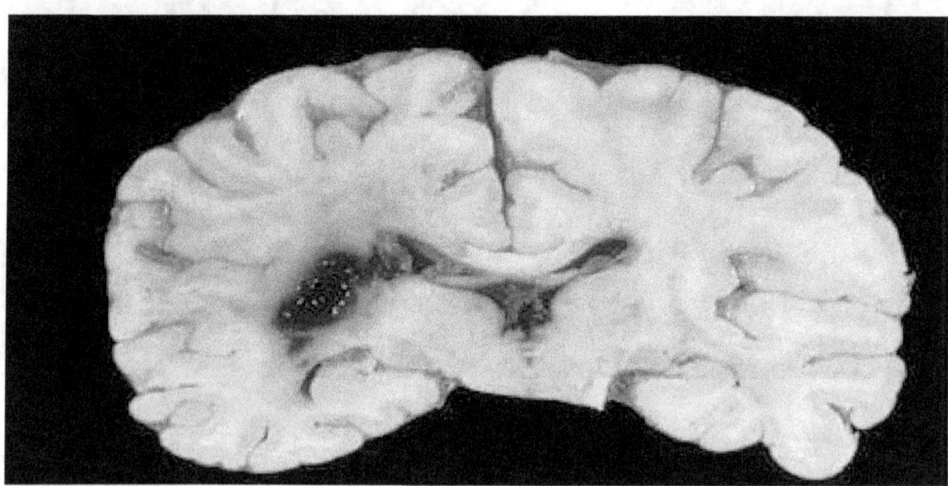

**14**

---

# SYMPTOM EIGHT

## BEING FRUSTRATED BY TASKS

Identifying brain damaged parts can relate to symptom eight.

**List of Brain Parts that Can Cause Symptom Eight Prefrontal cortex and Mediodorsal thalamus**

### 14.1 Neural representations of tasks

Neural representations of tasks and rules are maintained in the **prefrontal cortex,** the part of the brain responsible for planning action. Cognitive flexibility—the brain's ability to switch between different rules or action plans depending on the context is key to many of our everyday activities.

A new study from MIT has found that a region of the thalamus is key to the process of switching between the rules required for different contexts. This region, called the **mediodorsal thalamus,** suppresses representations that are not currently needed. That suppression also protects the representations as a short-term memory that can be reactivated when needed.

**Symptom Eight Diagnosis and Enhance MRI Imaging**

Even Mild COVID-19 May Change the Brain

**14.2 Prefrontal Cortex Thalamus**

MRI Diagnoses for Evidence of Previous Infection.

**Figure fifty-three: Previous COVID Infection Simple Image**

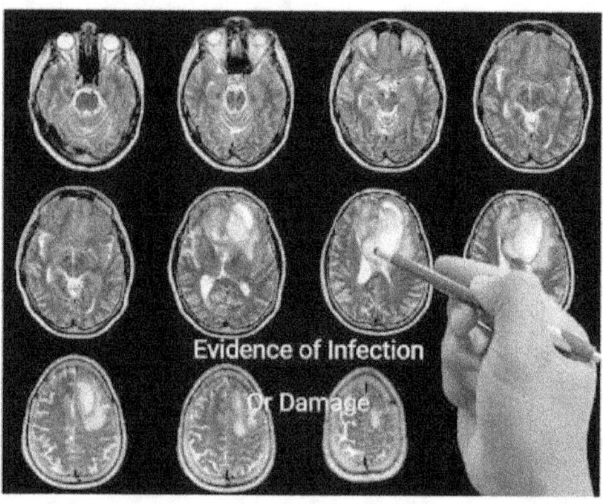


**Figure fifty-four: Thalamus Sample MRI Scan**

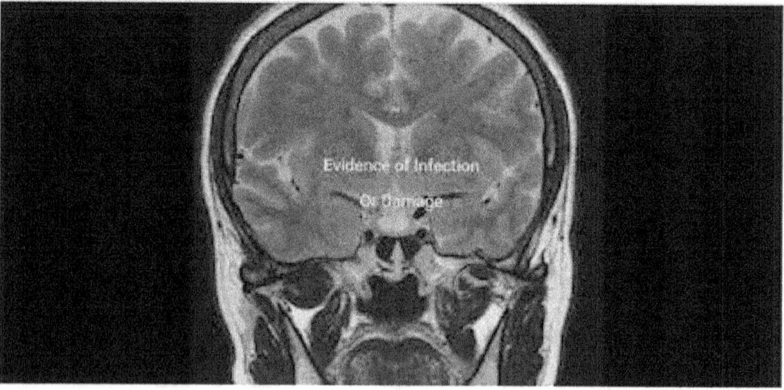

# Prefrontal Cortex Physical Location

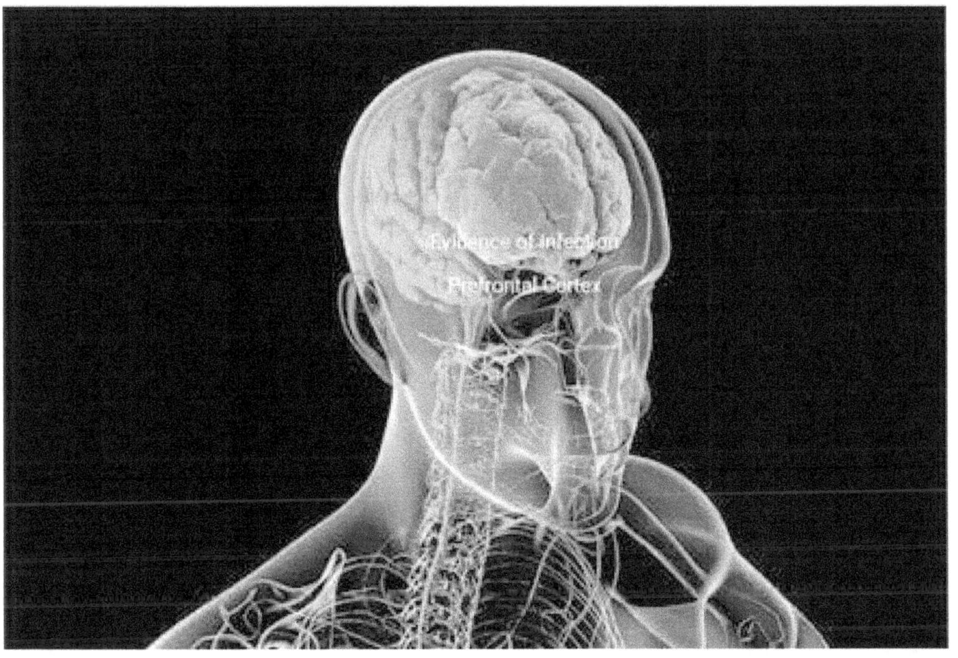

**15**

---

# SYMPTOM NINE

## ANXIETY IS OFTEN DRIVEN BY MANY FACTORS OTHER THAN POST COVID INFECTION

**Identifying brain damaged parts can relate to symptom nine.**

### 15.1 Anxiety and COVID-19

Coronavirus does not cause anxiety during the COVID infection. There is no study or specific damaged brain element indicating the cause of anxiety due to past infection.

### 15.2 Factors can trigger anxiety as:

1. Abuse. Physical, sexual, or emotional abuse can make you more vulnerable to depression later in life.
2. Age. People who are elderly are at higher risk of depression.
3. Certain medications
4. Conflict events
5. Death or the loss of a loved one
6. Gender
7. Genes
8. Work stress or job change

9. Change in living arrangements
10. Pregnancy and giving birth
11. Family and relationship problems
12. Major emotional shock following a stressful or traumatic event
13. Verbal, sexual, physical, or emotional abuse or trauma
14. Death or loss of a loved one

## 15.3 Common Triggers Related to post-COVID Infection

Research data shows almost 20 percent of people diagnosed with COVID-19 were then diagnosed with psychiatric disorders, including anxiety, depression, or insomnia. Meanwhile, COVID-19 itself can lead to neurological and mental complications, such as delirium, agitation, and stroke. People with preexisting mental, neurological, or substance use disorders are also more vulnerable to SARS-CoV-2 infection They may stand a higher risk of severe outcomes and even death.

**Figure fifty-five: No evidence of any brain damage is related to anxiety. Illustration.**

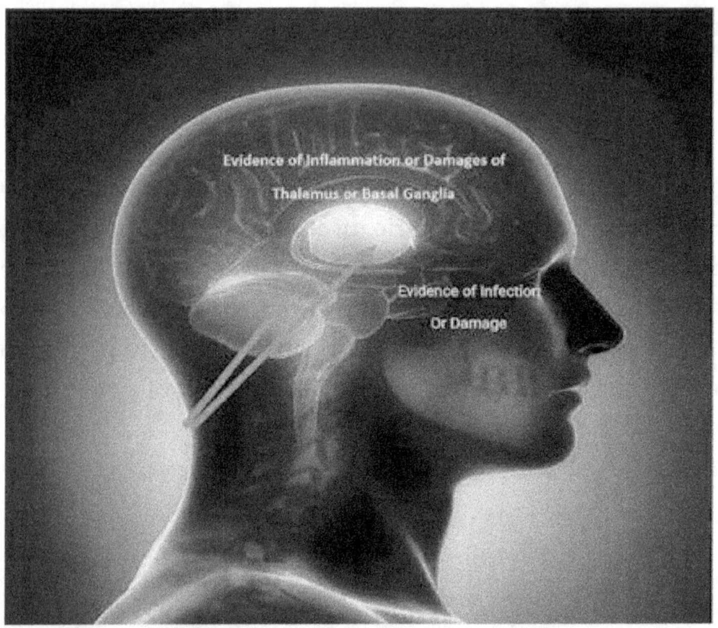


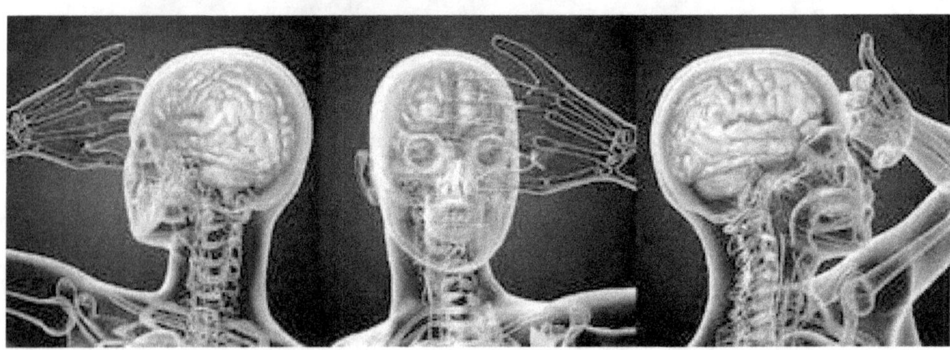

**16**

---

# SYMPTOM TEN

## FORGETTING TO DO THINGS OFTEN

**Identifying brain damaged parts can relate to symptom ten.**

### 16.1 Forgetfulness

It can arise from **stress, depression, lack of sleep or thyroid problems.** Other causes include side effects from certain medicines, an unhealthy diet or not having enough fluids in your body (dehydration). Taking care of these underlying causes may help resolve your memory problems

**List of Brain Parts that Can Cause Symptom Ten:** Frontal lobe of the cerebral cortex stored outside the Hippocampus

Short-term memory primarily takes place in the **frontal lobe of the cerebral cortex.** Then the information makes a stopover in the hippocampus.

This suggested that long-term episodic memories (memories of specific events) are stored **outside the hippocampus.** Scientists believe these memories are stored in the neocortex, the part of the brain also responsible for cognitive functions such as attention and planning.

## 16.2 Frontal lobe of the cerebral cortex

## Symptom Ten Diagnosis and Enhance MRI Imaging

## Figure fifty-six: Normal Brain MRI

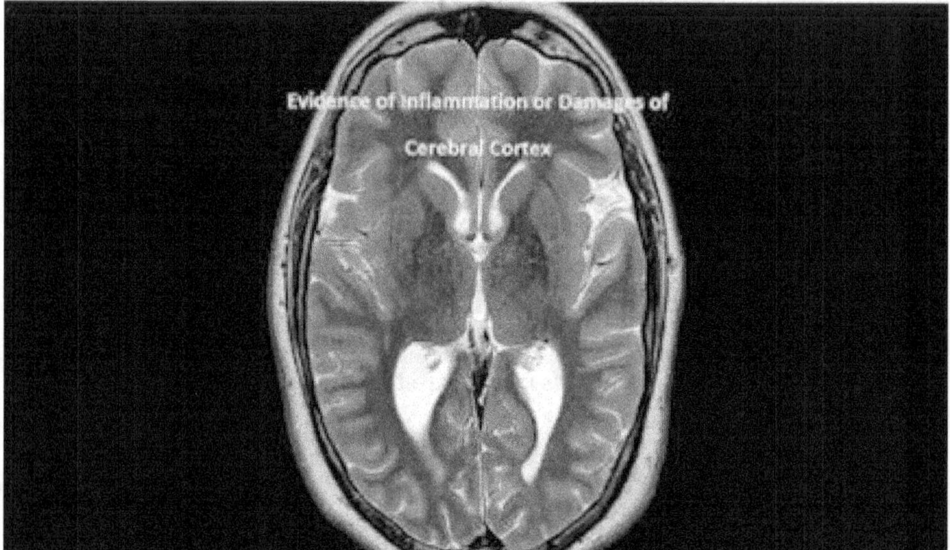


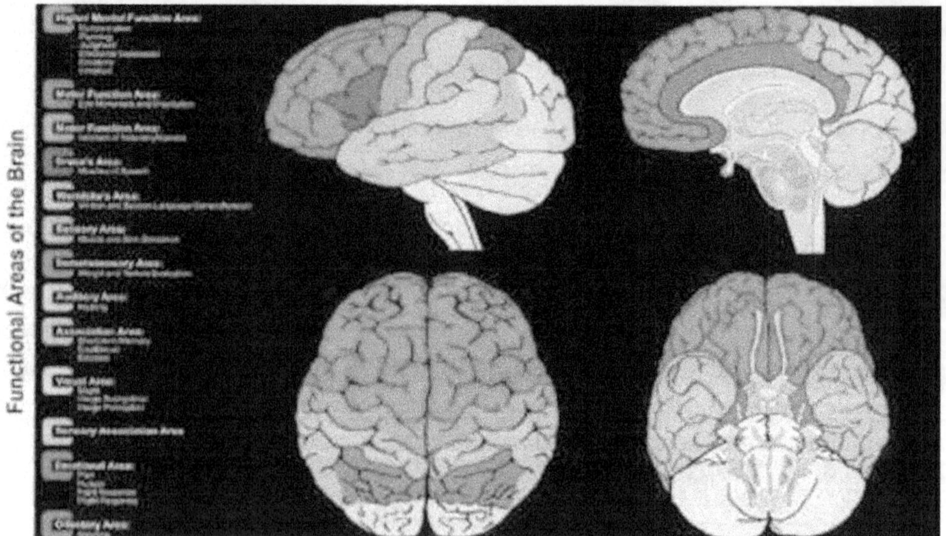

## 16.2.1 Doing tasks in the wrong order

Your **frontal lobes** are located right behind your forehead and are responsible for many functions that are vital for performing your daily activities.

## 16.3 Dementia damage showing in MRI Scan

**Figure fifty-seven: Advanced Dementia Sample Scan**

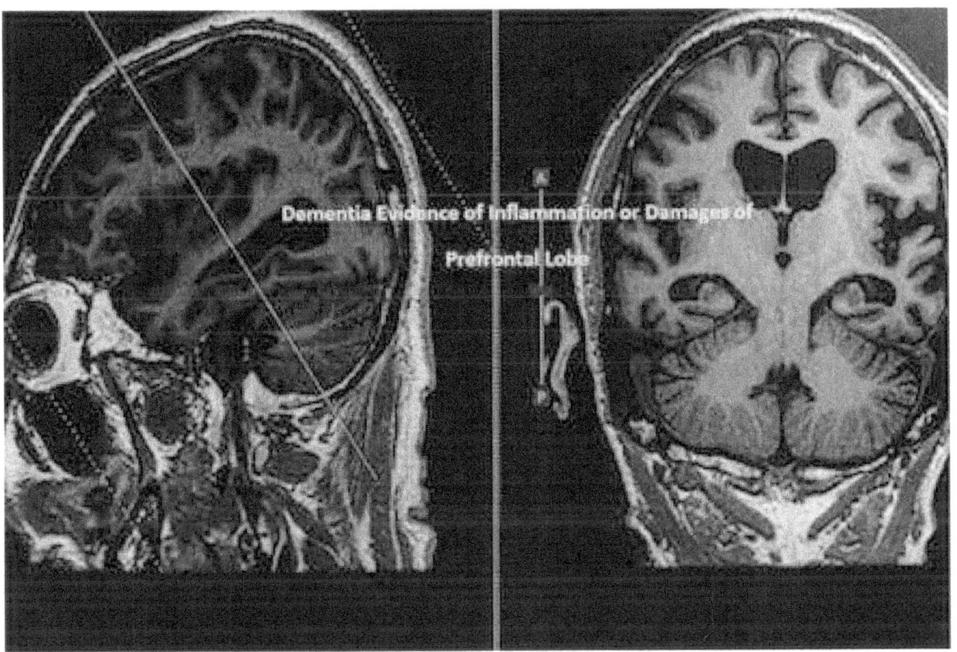

**17**

---

# SYMPTOM ELEVEN

## HEADACHE AND BEING UNCOMMUNICATIVE

**Identifying Brain Parts Damage Can Relates to Symptom Eleven**

**17.1 Brain Area of Investigation for being uncommunicative**

Recent research has revealed that contracting SARS-CoV-2, the virus that causes COVID-19, can have mental health problems. The study, published in The Lancet Psychiatry, analyzed the electronic health records of 69.8 million patients in the United States, which included 62,354 patients diagnosed with COVID-19. Within three months of testing positive, almost 20 percent of people diagnosed with COVID-19 were then diagnosed with psychiatric disorders, including anxiety, depression, or insomnia. One in four of those people had not received a psychiatric diagnosis before. The researchers warned that the results are likely to be underestimates of the actual number of cases.

**List of Brain Parts Can Cause Symptom Eleven:** Hypothalamic- pituitary adrenal and Blood Barrier Disruption as a Result of COVID Infection

Researchers found when you get infected with the virus that causes COVID-19, your <u>immune system</u> produces cytokines, chemokines, and other things that promote <u>inflammation</u>. Experts found that if your body doesn't properly control these cytokines, certain bad things can happen:

- Nerve inflammation
- <u>Blood</u> brain-barrier disruption
- Peripheral immune cell invasion into the <u>central nervous system</u>
- Impaired nerve transmission
- Hypothalamic-pituitary adrenal (HPA) axis dysfunction

**18**

---

# SYMPTOM TWELVE
## WORKING ON AUTOMATIC, NOT THINKING

**Identifying brain damaged parts can relate to symptom twelve.**

### 18.1 Brain Making Judgment

In brief, research on the unconscious mind has shown that **the brain makes judgments and decisions quickly and automatically.** It continuously makes predictions about future events. According to the theory of the "predictive mind," consciousness arises only when the brain's implicit expectations fail to materialize.

### 18.2 Having Difficulty Concentrating

You rely on concentration to get through work or school every day. When you're unable to concentrate, you can't think clearly, focus on a task, or maintain your attention. You may also find that you can't think as well, which can affect your decision-making. A few medical conditions may contribute to or cause inability to concentrate. There is no clear evidence that post- COVID infection can contribute to the symptoms. It's not always a medical emergency but being unable to concentrate can mean you need medical attention.

# SYMPTOM THIRTEEN
## VERTIGO BALANCE PROBLEM

**Identifying brain damaged parts can relate to symptom thirteen.**

### 19.1 Vertigo Caused by Post-COVID Infection

It is widely acknowledged that disorders that cause dizziness and vertigo are commonly caused by viral infections. Many of these infections can inflame and damage the inner ear (the vestibular organ) or other areas of the brain that coordinate motion and position, which can produce dizziness, nausea, imbalance, hearing issues and visual complaints.

The very high prevalence of the COVID-19 novel coronavirus and its variants means that millions of people are currently at risk of having issues with dizziness following infection.

Because COVID-19 causes inflammation in the nose and naso-pharynx (the upper part of the throat located behind the nose), the Eustachian tube (the tube that connects the nose and middle ear) may also become inflamed during the infection.

**List of Brain Parts that Can Cause Symptom Thirteen:** Vestibular Neuritis Nerve Damage

## 19.2 Vestibular Neuritis

Vestibular neuritis induced by COVID-19 is like any other **viral infection.** Whether in the inpatient or outpatient.

**Illustration: Feeling Imbalanced**

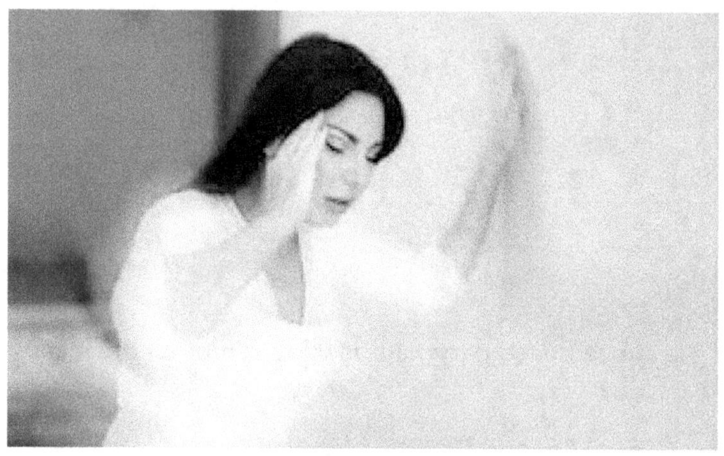

**Ilustration: Feeling Dizzy**

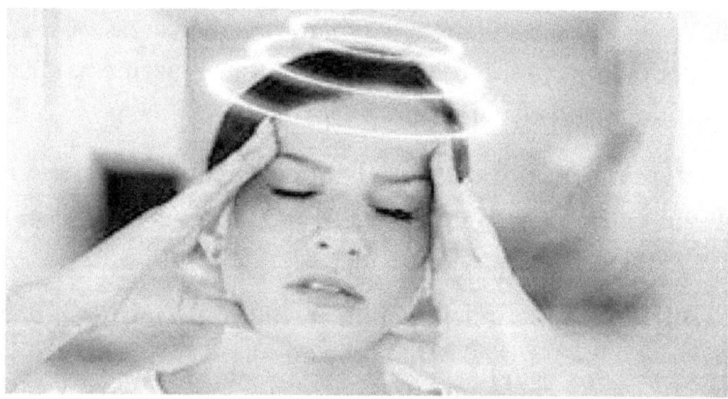

# Figure fifty-eight: Inner Ear Anatomy Illustration

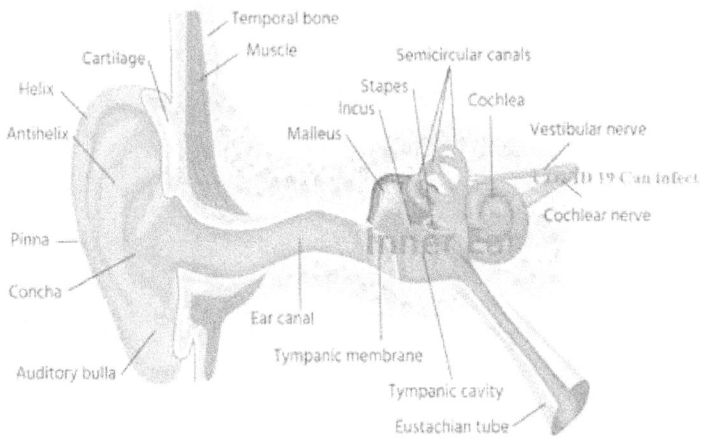



# Inner Ear Chrystal Alignment for Balance Regulation

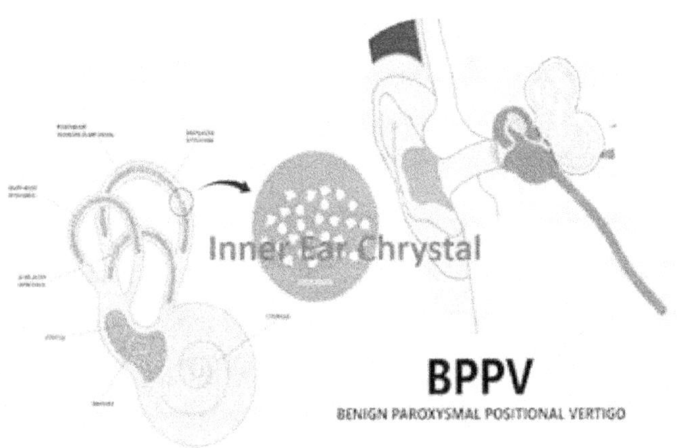



## 19.3 Vertigo vector illustration

Labeled medical vestibular ear problem scheme. Anatomical inner earlobe and canal detailed structure. Disease explanation with otoconia crystals disease comparison diagram.

**Figure fifty-nine: Vertigo Management**

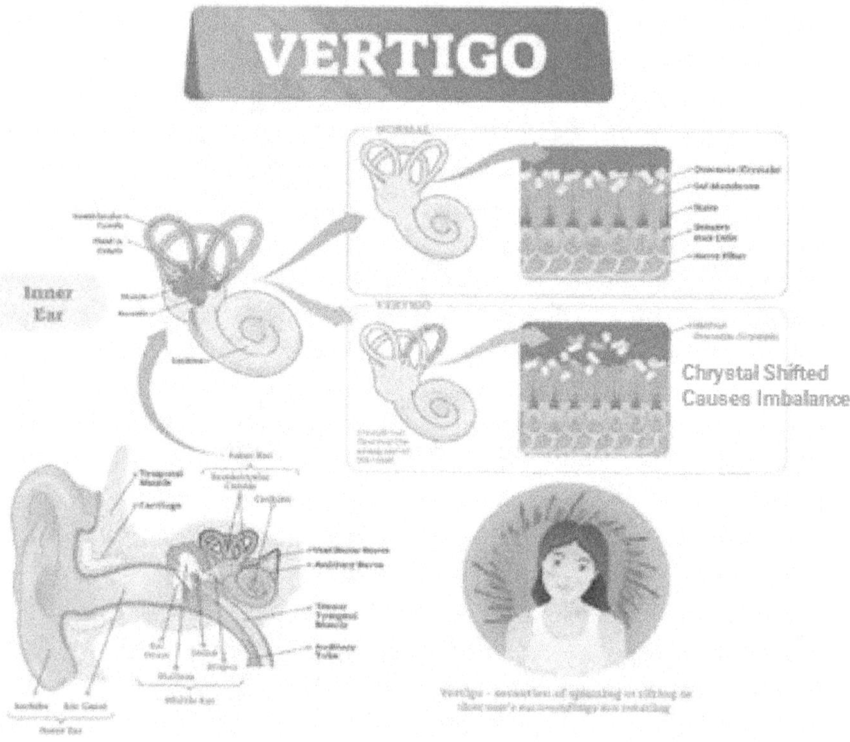


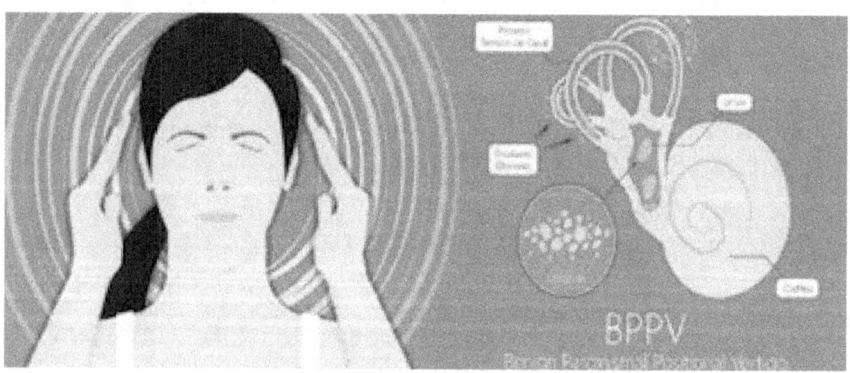

# Table eight: Summary of Brain Symptoms and Area of Diagnosis

| Managed Symptoms and Diagnosis | Examined Area of the Brain |
| --- | --- |
| **Symptom one**<br>Forgetting about Task started but did not get Completed | Brain frontal and temporal lobe for any cell's damages<br>Brain Cells Action Mass and Neurons |
| **Symptom Two**<br>Taking much longer than usual to complete simple tasks | Evidence of PFC Degradation<br>Prefrontal Cortex, the Prefrontal Cortex (PFC) and hippocampus are the most critical parts of the human brain for decision making |
| **Symptom Three**<br>Feeling frequently distracted | Prefrontal Cortex 32 & 24<br>Infarcted Areas |
| **Symptom Four**<br>Feeling tired when working | Diagnosis for Hypothalamus MRI Scan shows no any damages |
| **Symptom Five**<br>Needing more time to complete small task | Front Ganglia Examined<br>Limbic System |
| **Symptom Six**<br>Finding Difficulty Sleeping | Limbic System Pineal Gland and Hypothalamus. Evidence of any damages |
| **Symptom Seven**<br>Being more irritable than usual? | Examined<br>Amygdala and Limbic System |
| **Symptom Eight**<br>Being frustrated by tasks | Cerebral Cortex Infarct<br>Prefrontal Cortex Thalamus MRI Diagnosis for Evidence of Previous Infection or the Thalamus |
| **Symptom Nine**<br>A primary Other Disease by Mass Junction Other than Post COVID Infection | Evidence of Inflammation or Damage of Thalamus or Basal Ganglia |
| **Symptom Ten**<br>Forgetting to do things often | Frontal lobe of the cerebral cortex<br>Temporal lobe Infarct |
| **Symptom Eleven**<br>Headache and being unconcentrative | Hypothalamic-pituitary adrenal (HPA) axis dysfunction<br>Nerve inflammation<br>Blood-brain-barrier disruption |
| **Symptom Twelve**<br>Working on automatic not thinking | Hypothalamus Evidence of inflammation |
| **Symptom Thirteen**<br>Vertigo Balance Problems | Inner Ear<br>Vestibular neuritis induced by COVID-19 is like any other viral infection |
| **Symptom Fourteen**<br>How can COVID affect memory and thinking | Examined Hypothalamus and Prefrontal Lobe Neurons |

## 19.4 What are Post-COVID Dizziness Symptoms?

The long-haul symptoms associated with COVID 19 are varied and numerous. However, the most common symptoms related specifically to dizziness and vestibular issues are:

- Generalized dizziness. Some report feeling "drunk or tipsy" without having any alcohol.
- Lightheadedness or a floating feeling

- Vertigo or a spinning sensation, particularly when looking up or down, or lying on your side
- Poor balance when standing or changing positions
- Problems walking in a straight line or in busy areas such as a shopping mall
- Nausea or vomiting

## 19.5 Understanding General Causes Of Dizziness And Imbalance

Dizziness is usually diagnosed as either:

1. a problem WITH your vestibular system
2. a problem OUTSIDE of your vestibular system

Your vestibular system allows you to sense movement accurately and lets you react properly to motion and changes in position. It consists of vestibular organ in your inner ear, and the areas of your brain that process vestibular information and the vestibular nerves that connect these two areas.

Problems WITH your vestibular system are one of the most common reasons for dizziness. Affected areas can include the inner ear, the brain, the vestibular nerves, or any combination of those structures.

### 19.5.1 How does COVID-19 cause dizziness?

The coronavirus disease has been shown to cause organ complica- tions due to inflammatory reactions. For example, the inflammation of the heart and lungs cause some of the classic post-COVID symp- toms such as breathing difficulties, coughing, and chronic fatigue. Inflammation of our inner ear and vestibular centers of the brain can quickly create a range of dizziness related symptoms.

## 19.6 When Does Dizziness From Long COVID Start?

Dizziness is a common feature of COVID infection, and in many patients, the dizziness symptoms begin at the time of initial infec- tion. However, typical spinning type of dizziness (vertigo) that is associated with sudden onset acute attacks of the vestibular system will usually present earlier after infection, often within the first week.

Imbalance and dizziness that is non-spinning can start occurring weeks after contraction of COVID-19. In these cases, the effects of the coronavirus on the vestibular system and other body systems can combine and become more apparent as your body continues its struggle, fighting the longer-term effects of the virus post-COVID.

## 19.6 Dizziness And Vertigo After COVID-19 Vaccination

All vaccinations (and medical interventions in general) come with some risk of adverse side-effects, including COVID-19 vaccinations such as with Pfizer/Bio-NTech, AstraZeneca, and Moderna. Vaccine surveillance reports do indicate that vertigo, tinnitus, and hearing loss are a small part of the group of possible symptoms related to post-vaccination side effects. However, more studies are needed to determine the nature of this relationship and any long-term symptoms and consequences.

On a positive note, it has been observed that the majority of those who find any symptoms of dizziness after vaccination find them mild and temporary.

**20**

---

# MANAGING VERTIGO

20.1 Differentiate between old age Vertigo and vestibular neuritis

What causes vestibular neuritis? Researchers think the most likely cause is **a viral infection of the inner ear, swelling around the ves- tibulocochlear nerve (caused by a virus), or a viral infection that has occurred somewhere else in the body.**

Reports on lower motor neuron facial palsy or **vestibular neuritis** are sparse by the virus entering the cell using **ACE-2 receptors** and infecting healthy cells.

**20.2 Treatment Of Vestibular Neuronitis Physician Recommendation Is Advised**

- Drugs such as meclizine or lorazepam to relieve vertigo.
- Drugs such as prochlorperazine to relieve vomiting.
- Sometimes corticosteroid drugs such as prednisone.
- Intravenous fluids if vomiting persists.
- Physical therapy.
- Treatment and cure should be decided by the patient's physician only.

**21**

---

# HOW CAN COVID AFFECT MEMORY AND THINKING

Memory: if your memory is affected, you may find it difficult to hold information in your head to use it to make decisions based on that information. You may struggle to recall something that has happened, or forget to take medication on time.

Attention and concentration: problems with attention/concentra- tion can make it hard to focus and ignore distractions and not be distracted when trying to concentrate on a task.

Brain executive functions are the mental processes that allow us to solve problems, make decisions, plan, and see tasks through to completion.

For example, executive functions are needed to deal with problems, organize a holiday, get

People with executive functioning problems often seem disorganized, impulsive, and not thinking things through. They may find it difficult to get going on tasks.

The hypothalamus holds the executive function of the brain to per- form and organize tasks. Refer to the previous section of this book for brain limbic system imaging.

**22**

---

# SYMPTOMS: QUESTIONS AND ANSWERS

## 22.1 Why Does COVID Affect Memory and Thinking?

There are several reasons why people who have been ill with COVID might experience difficulties in their memory and thinking skills. Related to the following:

### 22.1.1 Fatigue

Fatigue is common after viral infections and can affect your ability to concentrate. You may feel that you don't have the mental energy needed to pay attention to things, even when you think something is important. If you can't concentrate on something, it is harder to remember it. If you have returned to work, it may be difficult to concentrate on work tasks.

### 22.1.1 Fear and Anxiety

The COVID pandemic has been a worrying time, and for some people, it may have caused high levels of anxiety and even panic attacks. Recovering from COVID can be a stressful experience for many people, whether this was at home or within a hospital setting.

### 22.1.3 Low mood

Low mood can affect memory and thinking. During the COVID pandemic, many people have faced situations that may have become overwhelming and led to low mood. Like anxiety, low mood affects the ability to concentrate and remember things.

### 22.2 Brain inflammation

In a small number of people, COVID causes inflammation in the brain. If this was the case, your team of health care professionals would have told you that tests showed evidence of brain inflammation known as encephalitis; its effects depend on which parts of the brain have been affected. These often include difficulties with attention/ concentration and memory.

# 23

## MANAGING NEUROLOGICAL PROBLEMS

### 23.1 Managing Attention and Concentration Problems

If your attention capacity is limited, it can be very helpful to reduce distractions. If you are trying to do something demanding, like fill out a complicated form, find a time and place that is quiet and ask others around you not to disturb you. You might also find listening to gentle instrumental music helps.

### 23.1.1 Managing Memory Problems

If you find that you have problems remembering to do things, or if you struggle to remember things you have done or information you've been told, then it can really help to use an external aid to share the load. To remember to do things, you can use your phone's calendar app to automatically remind you when you must do things.

### 23.1.2 Managing Executive Problems

Setting up a regular routine that works well for you will reduce the demands on your brain. Think through all the things you want to regularly do every day, or every week, put them into a schedule, and practice this routine until it becomes second nature.

Make a clear plan before approaching any new or complicated problem or situation, break the problem down into all the steps you need to take, write each one down and what you need for it, and then follow it. Keep checking back to your plan to check you haven't gone off course and to check if you need to change your plan.

**24**

---

# WHEN YOU NEED TO SEE A DOCTOR

**24.1 What signs should someone look out for? And when should they go to a doctor about brain fog?**

Symptoms like weakness, difficulty speaking, loss of vision, numb- ness, and tingling indicate that there's damage in one part of the nervous system. There could be dysfunction of the nerve cells in the brain without us seeing anything on the MRI imaging. And that could be due to inflammation in neurotransmit- ters molecules that allow nerve cells to talk to each other and not be func- tioning normally as related to post-COVID-19 infections.

# Patients Information Survey
## Discovery of any Previous COVID 19 Infection

**Patient Information Survey**

Patient Name ________________________ Age ________________

Patient Home Address ______________________________________________

Did you Receive Vaccine: Pfizer        Modena        J&J

When did you receive vaccine ________________________

Did you get infected with COVID 19        When ________________

Asymptomatic ________ Mild Symptoms ____________ Sever Symptoms ____________

Have you been hospitalized ____________________

Supervised Medication Administered ________________________________

Period Spent in hospital ____________________

Time discharged from the hospital ____________________

**Please Check the Symptom That Applied to You**

| | Yes | No | Explanation of Persistent Symptom |
|---|---|---|---|

**25**

---

# BRAIN ANATOMY REFERENCE DIAGRAMS

**Diagram A1: Human Brain Diagram**

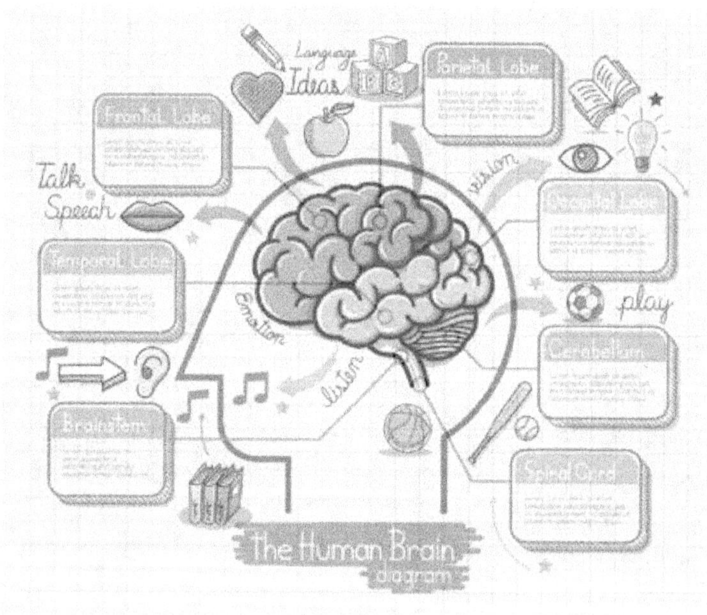

# Diagram A2: Median Section of the BrainDiagram

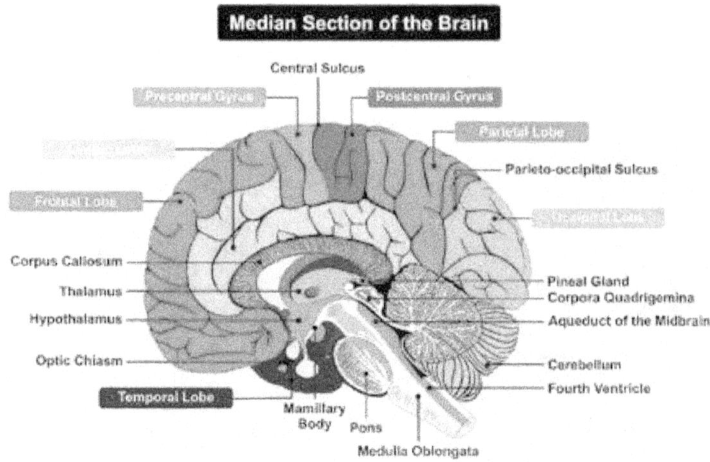


# Diagram A3: Brain Nucleus

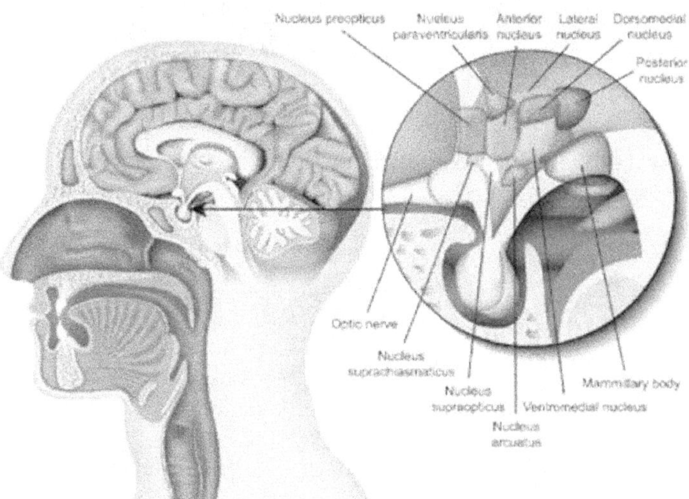


What is the brain nucleus?

These deep brain structures together largely control voluntary skeletal move-ment. The caudate nucleus functions not only in planning the execution of movement but also in learning, memory, reward, motivation, emotion, and romantic interaction.


## Diagram A4: Brain High Mental Function

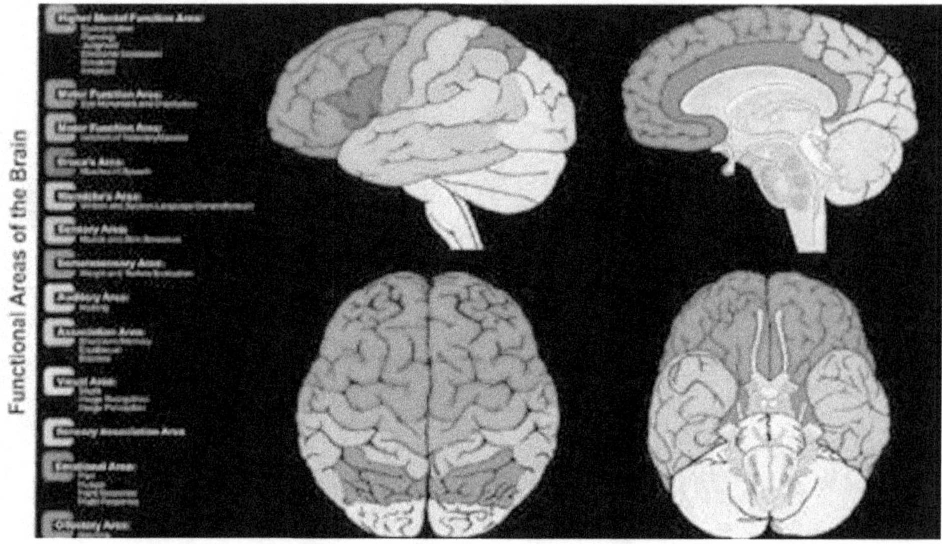



## A5: Brain Concentration and Planning

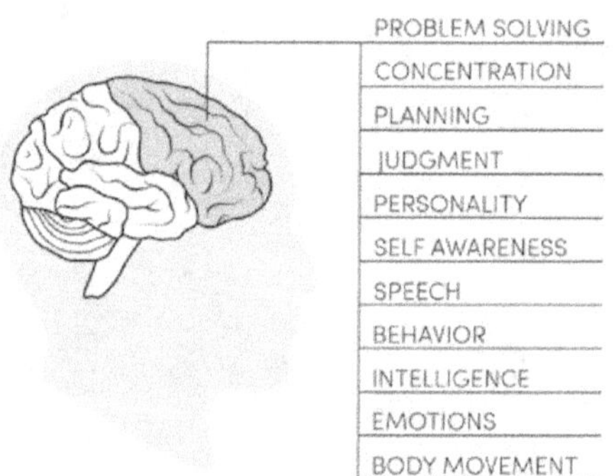

## Diagram A6: Brain Sulcus and Gyrus Diagram

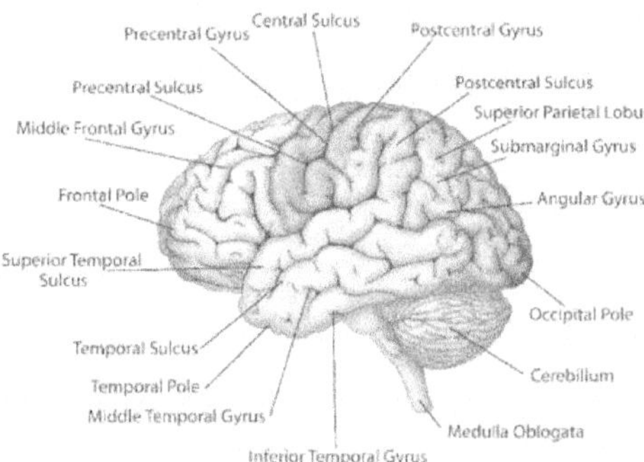


## What is the brain sulcus and gyrus?

Each gyrus is surrounded by sulci, and together, the gyri and sulci **help to increase the surface area of the cerebral cortex and form brain divisions.** They form brain divisions by creating boundaries between the lobes, so these are easily identifiable, as well as serving to divide the brain into two hemispheres.

# Diagram A7: Brain Nerve System

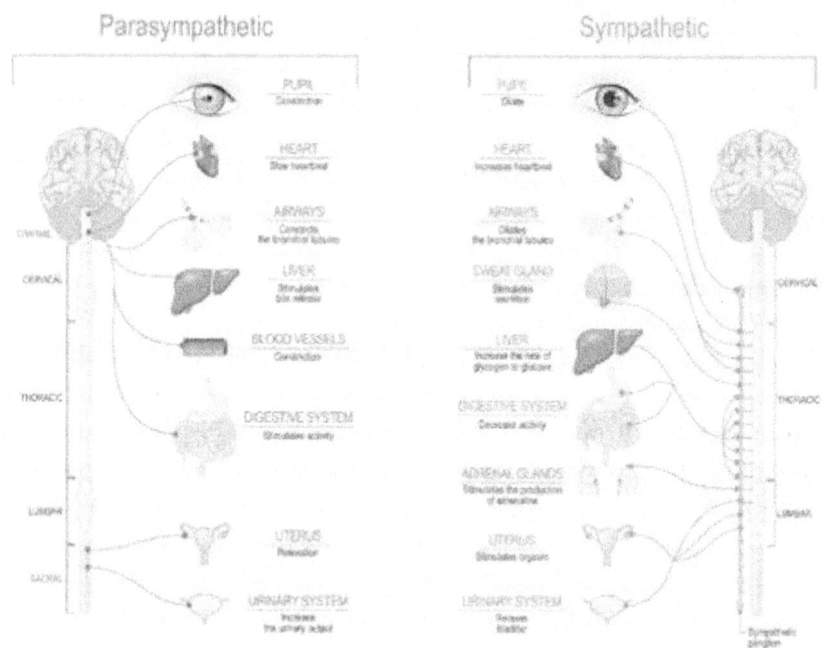



# Diagram A8: Brain MRI Lobes Infarct

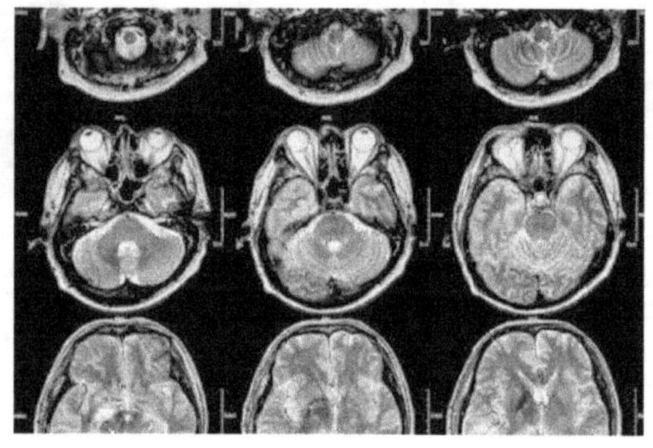

# Diagram A9: Brain Detailed Synaptic

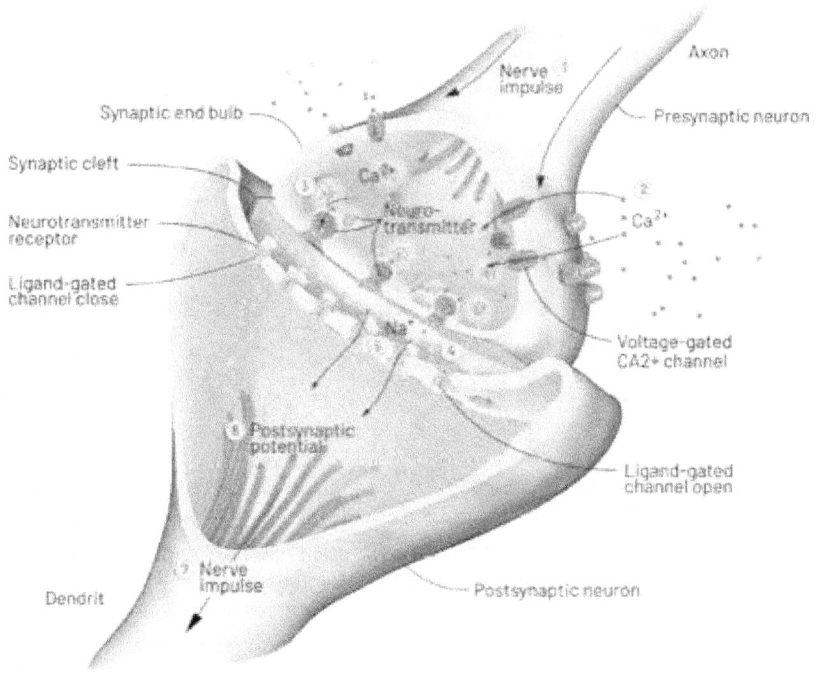

# Diagram A10: Brain Neuron Communication

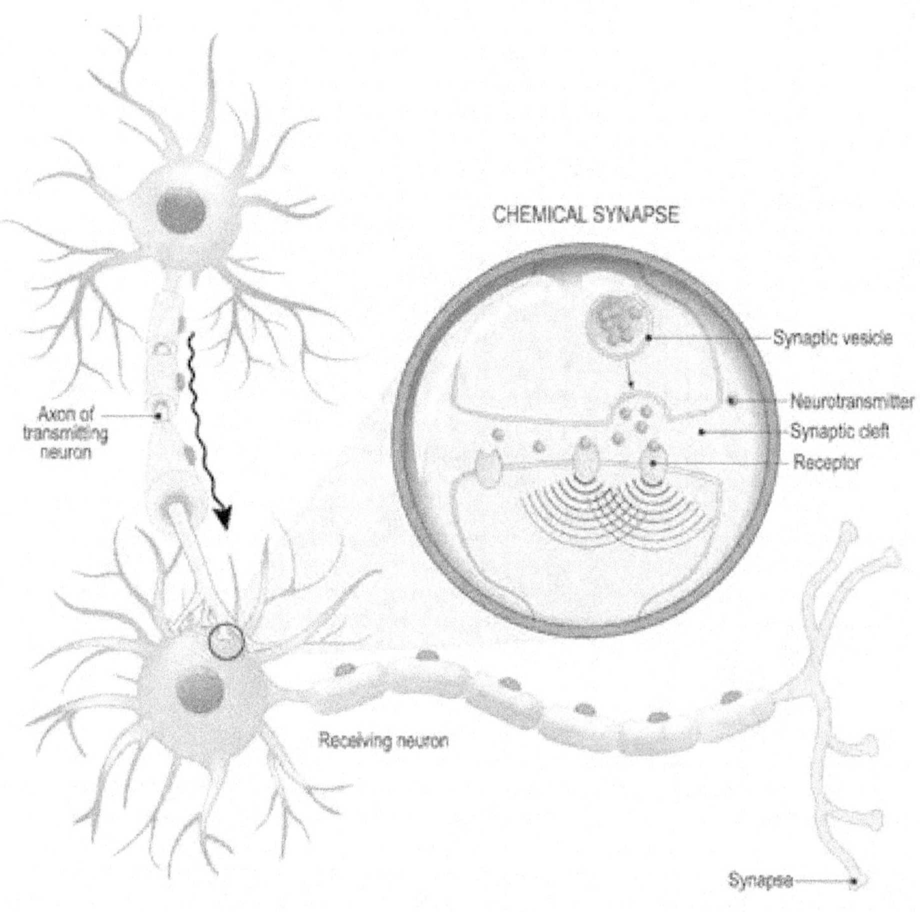

## Diagram A11: Brain Left and Right Function

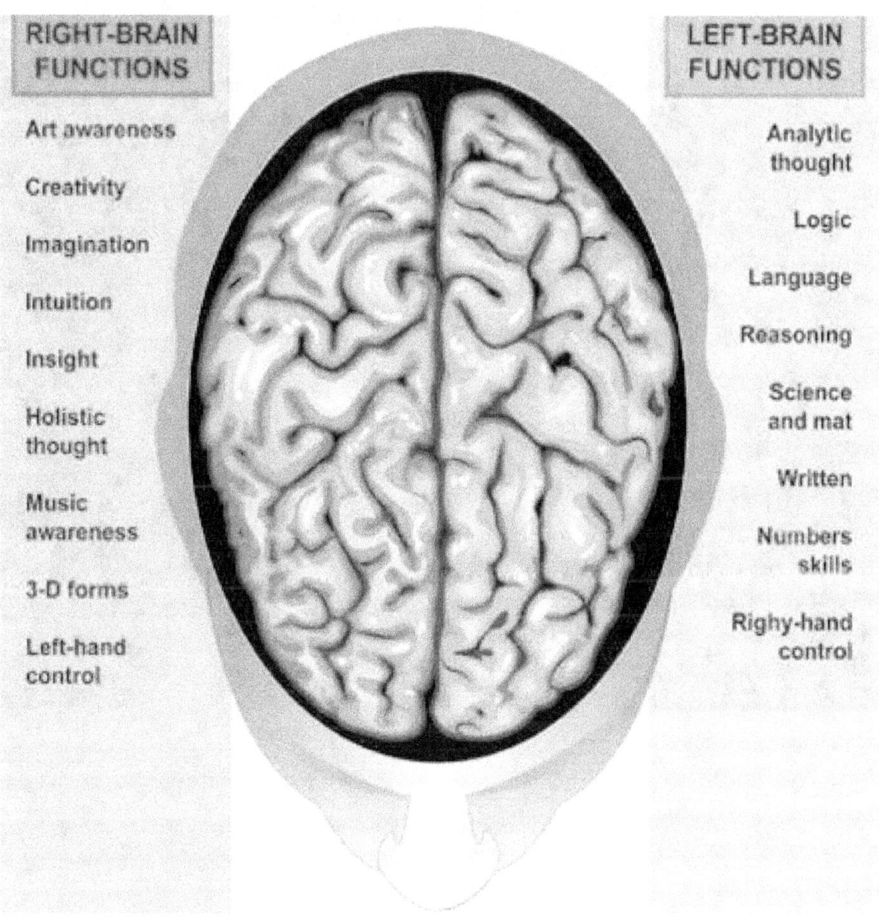

# Diagram A12: Limbic System Physical Location

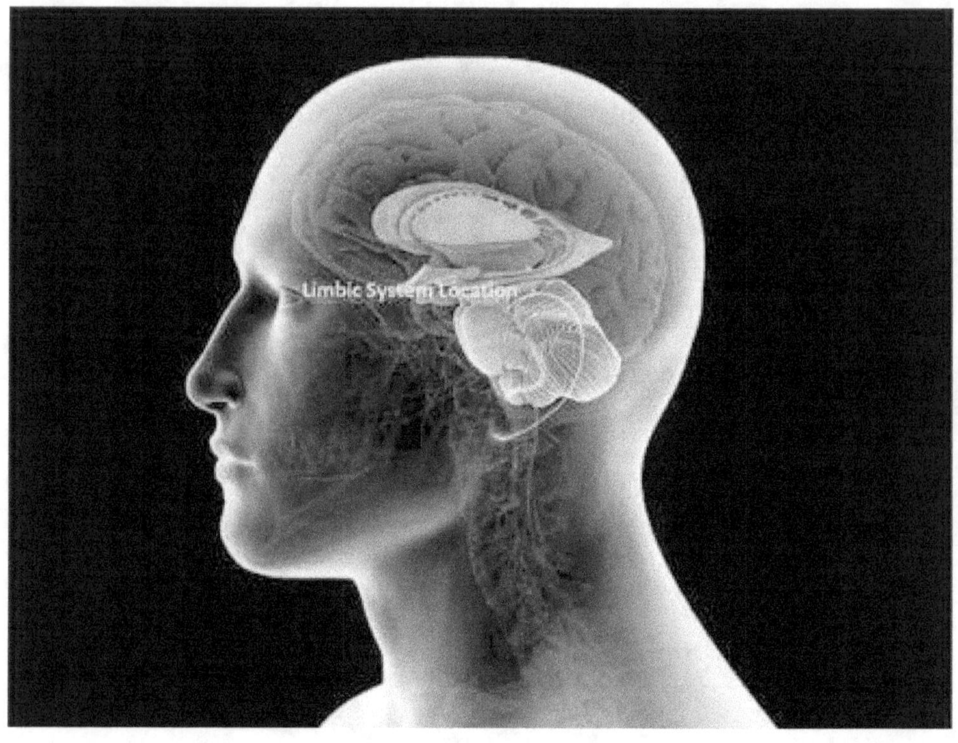

**Diagram A13: Brain Blood Supply Showing Arteries Blood Clots**

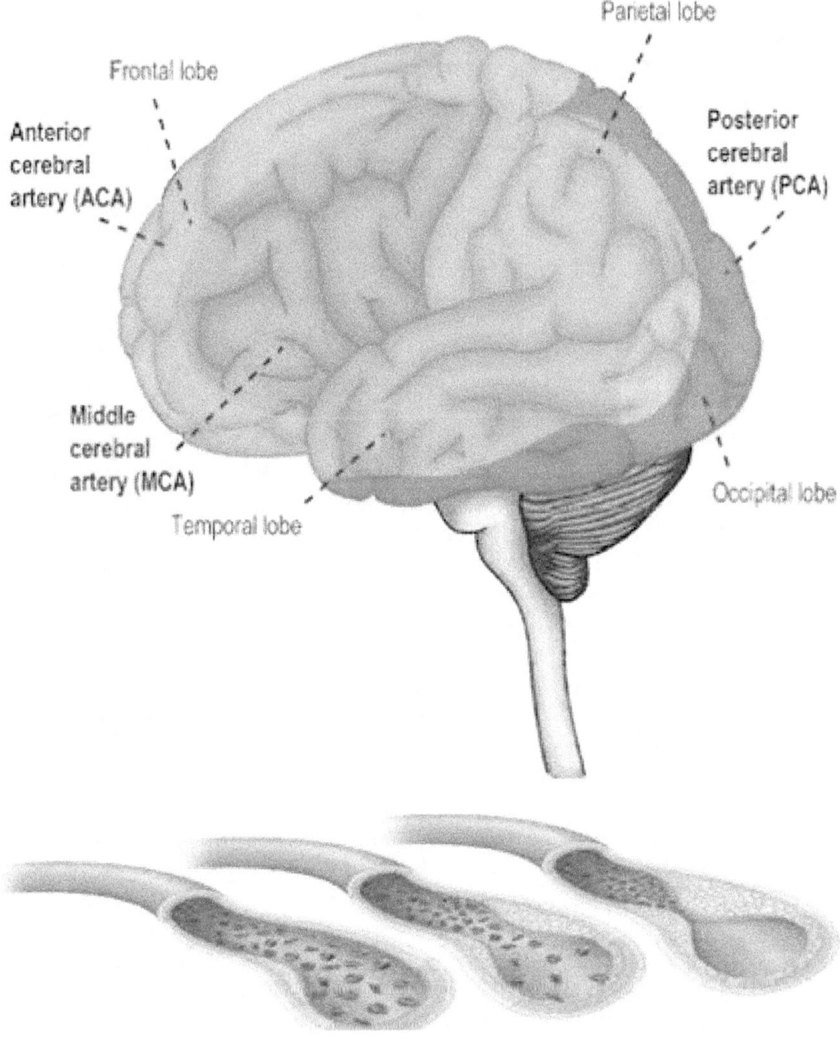

## Diagram A14: Brain Peripheral Nerve System

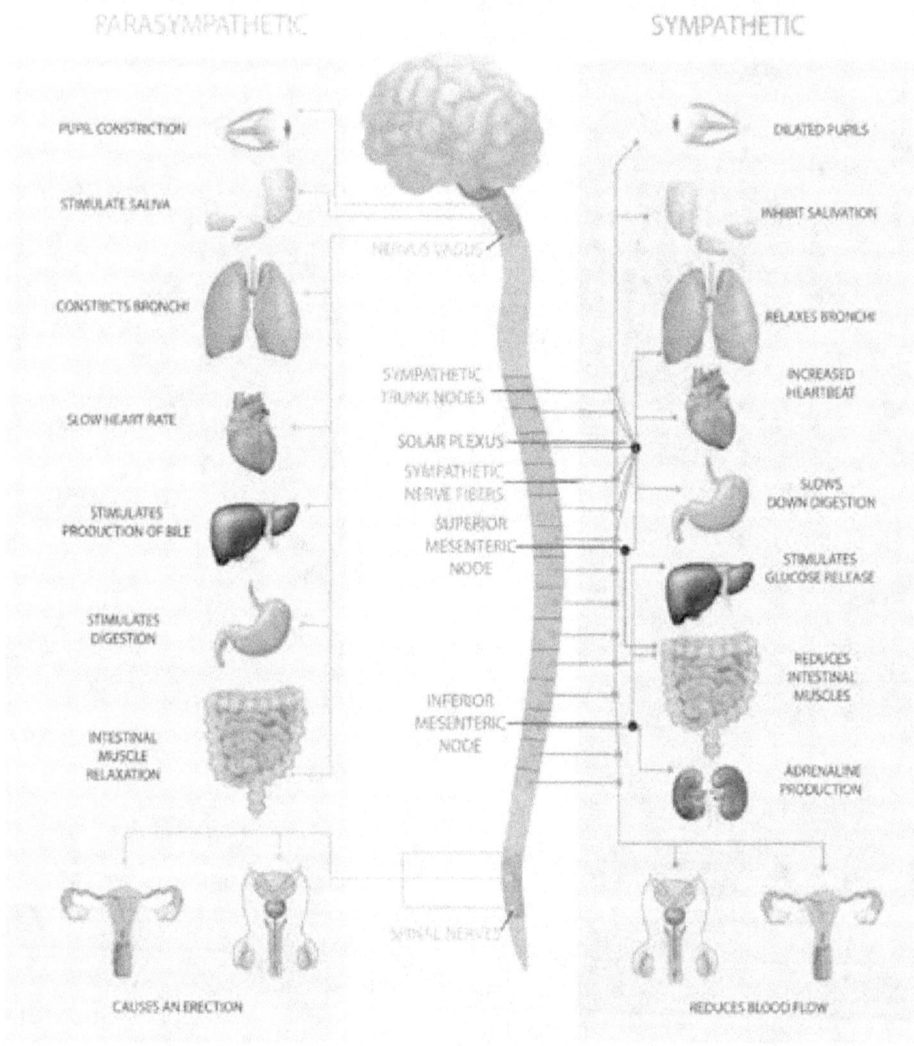

**Diagram A15: Brain Neuron Anatomy**

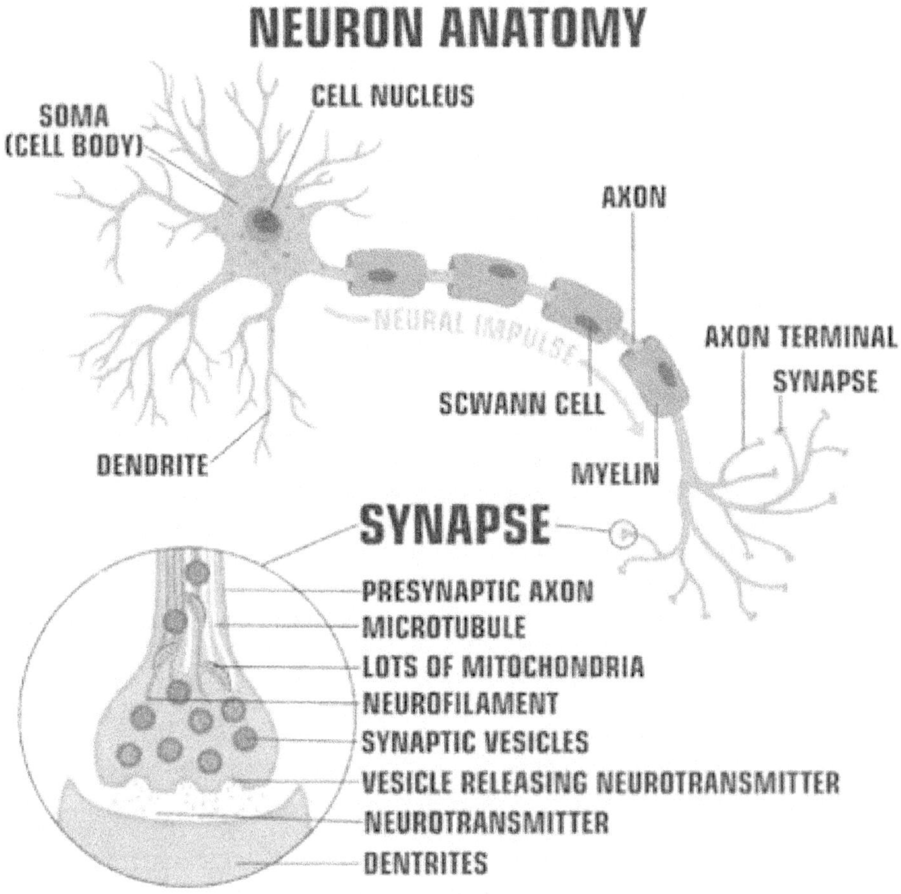

# Synaptic transmission

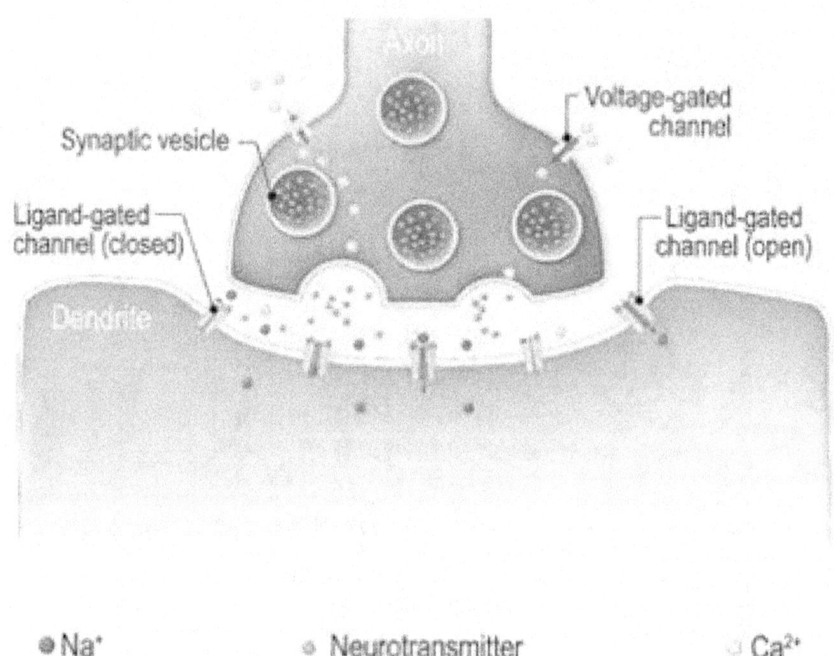

**26**

---

# OTHER POST-COVID-19 SYMPTOMS RELATED TO DIFFERENT ORGANS

**26.1 Other Post-COVID-19 symptoms are broken down into the following categories:**

A Cardiovascular system-related symptoms

B Respiratory system-related symptoms

C Liver-related symptoms

D Renal-related symptoms

E Gastrointestinal system-related symptoms

F Endocrine systems-related symptoms

G Lymphatics system-related symptoms

**26.2 List of identified post-COVID-19 symptoms from trusted scientific sources for information only**

**Note:** Some of these symptoms are still under investigation and clinical research and can relate to other chronic illnesses rather than post-COVID infection. All listed information in this section is credited to the originator, and I claim no ownership or rights to the listed information.

These symptoms listing reported during the infection and others as Long Hauler.

1. **Elevated thyroid:** Some COVID-19 sufferers report having elevated thyroid levels as a long-lasting symptom of the virus.
2. **Anemia: Anemia** is "a condition in which you lack enough healthy red blood cells to carry adequate oxygen to your body's tissues," says the Mayo Clinic. The most common type of anemia is associated with not getting enough iron. The condition makes you feel tired and weak. In some cases, it may even cause chest pain and dizziness, which are common long-lasting symptoms of COVID-19.
3. **Symptoms of herpes:** Epstein-Barr Virus (EBV) and trigeminal neuralgia are varied and may include fatigue, inflamed throat, fever, and facial pain. These are also common symptoms of COVID-19, and thirty-eight sufferers who participated in the survey reported experiencing symptoms of these conditions after the virus was gone.
4. **GERD: It is acid reflux,** and it's commonly known to cause excessive salivation or drooling. According to the University of Florida Health, trauma or infections in the throat, such as sinus infections or swollen adenoids, can cause GERD, which may lead to drooling.
5. **Personality changes:** Scientists are studying the rare but potentially severe personality changes that COVID-19 may cause in patients. According to an article published in *Science News*, symptoms related to the brain are often overlooked as medical professionals focus on the physical aspects of the virus. However, depression, personality changes, and confusion are some long-lasting symptoms that some COVID-19 sufferers may experience.
6. **Thrush:** They are small white lesions inside your mouth caused by an imbalance of bacterial growth, more specifically an overgrowth of candida, according to Cedars-Sinai. Some people are more prone to developing thrush, but it may also be common with COVID-19 survivors.

7. **Hormonal imbalance:** Hormones are important because they regulate your appetite, mood, sexual function, and body temperature. According to Women in Balance Institute, a hormone imbalance may be caused by stress, an unhealthy lifestyle, or a buildup of toxins in the body. COVID-19 sufferers may experience this imbalance as the virus wreaks havoc on their respiratory system and as their immune system works hard to fight it off.

8. **Urinary tract infection:** Occurs when germs get into the urethra and begin to spread throughout the urinary tract, says John Hopkins Medicine. One study published in Elsevier Public Health Emergency Collection "found a potentially dangerous overlap of classical urinary symptoms and the as yet not fully described symptoms of COVID- 19." Urinary frequency and the virus may be related, which explains its potential cause of UTIs in patients.

9. **Kidney issues:** Kidney issues, including protein in the urine, were long-lasting symptoms of COVID-19 for for twenty-seven survey participants. The specific ways the virus affects kidneys isn't known yet, but according to John Hopkins Medicine, it may invade kidney cells, or the low levels of oxygen the virus causes may be what contribute to these long-lasting kidney problems.

10. **Dry scalp and dandruff:** Can be uncomfortable and embarrassing. According to Cedars-Sinai, dandruff can be caused by changes in hormones, so it makes sense that it's related to the virus.

11. **Low blood pressure:** According to the Mayo Clinic, low blood pressure is also related to infections and hormone fluctuations, which is why it may be a long-lasting symptom of COVID-19.

12. **COVID toes:** An emerging symptom of the virus that may not be as common as the other symptoms such as cough or fever. COVID toes occur when the toes developed a rash or lesions. According to Dr. Humberto Choi MD, from the Cleveland Clinic, rashes on the skin are common with viral infections such as COVID-19. The survey found that fifty-nine participants had this strange side effect after being infected with coronavirus.

13. **Eye infection:** According to the University of Miami, it's possible that coronavirus could cause an eye infection, such as conjunctivitis, also

known as pink eye. The American Academy of Ophthalmology concludes that styes are caused by bacterial infections, which could explain the relationship between this eye condition and the virus.

14. **Foot pain:** Can be caused by a number of ailments, such as corns, plantar fasciitis, or Achill's tendon injury. "COVID toes" may contribute to this pain since some patients can have trouble walking or sleeping due to lesions on their toes. In most cases, this strange symptom goes away, so the foot pain should also subside.

15. **Goiter: An "abnormal enlargement of the thyroid gland,"** according to the American Thyroid Association. While a goiter doesn't necessarily mean the thyroid isn't functioning correctly, it does indicate that there's a potential hormonal imbalance causing the thyroid gland to grow abnormally. Seventy survey respondents dealt with a goiter after COVID-19, possibly due to the hormonal effects the virus has on the body.

16. **Cracked or dry lips:** Can occur in especially cold or hot weather, or maybe a sign of dehydration. When a virus like COVID-19 takes hold, dry lips may also occur because viruses are likely to cause dehydration. The American Academy of Dermatology suggests using lip balm, drinking plenty of fluids, and refraining from picking at the dry skin to get this symptom to go away.

17. **COVID-19 is a respiratory virus,** so it's no wonder those who contracted the illness feel a cold or burning sensation in their lungs. However, this symptom may last longer than the virus since seventy-four survey participants reported this feeling after the coronavirus was gone. An article published in *NBC News* concludes that many COVID-19 sufferers felt this "slow burn" for a while until it either worsened and was treated or went away completely.

18. **Bluish lips:** According to the Centers for Diseases Control and Prevention (CDC), bluish lips or face is an emergency of COVID-19. When your lips turn blue, it's a sign your blood oxygen has dipped to extreme levels. The survey found that seventy-seven participants claimed they experienced low blood oxygen after contracting coronavirus.

19. **Arrhythmia: Mayo** Clinic defines arrhythmia as a heart rhythm problem and explains it happens when "electrical impulses that coordinate your heartbeats don't worry properly, causing your heart to beat too fast, too slow or irregularly." A study published in Heart Rhythm studied hospitalized coronavirus patients and found some of them suffered bradyarrhythmia or cardiac arrests. The study concluded heart traumas and abnormalities like these are "likely the consequence of systemic illness and not solely the direct effects of COVID-19 infection."

20. **Jaw pain:** In the survey, eighty participants reported jaw pain as a long-lasting symptom of COVID-19. According to the American Dental Association, jaw pain may be caused by bone problems, stress, infection, sinus issues, or tooth grinding. It's known that coronavirus causes aches and pains, so this jaw pain may be a lingering side effect of the body fighting off the virus.

21. **Painful scalp:** For COVID-19 sufferers, a painful scalp may be a side effect of the dandruff the virus may cause, or aches and pains associated with the illness. According to Kaiser Permanente, scalp pain or ailments may occur after recovering from a high fever, when dealing with a thyroid issue, or if you have poor nutrition.

22. **Fizzing sensation:** According to an article published in St. Peter's Health Partners, a "tingling, burning, or 'fizzing' sensation" was reported from several COVID-19 patients. This sensation may be a side effect of other symptoms, such as aches and pains or fever.

23. **Back pain:** According to the National Institute of Neurological Disorders and Stroke, back pain intensity can range "from a dull, constant ache to a sudden, sharp or shooting pain." Those recovering from illness may report this pain due to a decrease in movement over the past few days or due to the usual aches and pains of their sickness. Eighty-four survey respondents claimed middle-back pain or gain at the base of their ribs after COVID-19. It's usually treated with muscle relaxants, gentle stretching, heat, or ice.

24. **Low temperature:** After potentially experiencing a fever while fighting off COVID-19, sufferers may be surprised by the strange long-lasting symptom of a low body temperature once they've recovered. According

to Kaiser Permanente, a low body temperature may occur with an infection, or maybe a sign of diabetes or a low thyroid level. A low temperature may also be the culprit for chills, since the body attempts to warm up with narrowed blood vessels.

25. **Your veins circulate** the blood around your body, and when you're too cold or hot, your blood vessels may constrict or widen. This may be due to having a fever, then low body temperature, or it may be a sign of dehydration. According to the Mayo Clinic, these bulging veins may be due to inactivity or damaged blood valves.

26. **Arthralgia (joint pain)** is a common symptom of coronavirus, and a study published in the Nature Public Health Emergency Collection found that at least one patient in the forty that were studied experienced joint pain. This joint ailment may linger in those who had the virus, causing hand or wrist pain to remain

27. **Costochondritis:** Mayo Clinic defines costochondritis as "inflammation of the cartilage that connects a rib to the breastbone (sternum)." Cedars-Sinai claims that the risk of developing a chest wall infection like costochondritis is increased with respiratory trauma, such as pneumonia or bronchitis. Since COVID-19 is a respiratory illness, it's not surprising that ninety-eight survey respondents who had the virus claimed costochondritis as a lingering symptom.

28. **Spike in blood pressure:** According to Rush University Medical Center, a spike in blood pressure could be caused by several factors, such as stress, thyroid problems, or certain medications. A study published by the American College of Cardiology found a potential link between the virus: the renin-angiotensin-aldosterone system, which is a "critical neurohormonal pathway that regulates blood pressure and fluid balance." This may explain the changes in blood pressure these patients experienced after coronavirus.

29. **Kidney problems:** According to the National Kidney Foundation, acute kidney damage occurs in about fifteen percent of COVID-19 patients, some of which never had kidney problems before. The survey found that 115 respondents have kidney pain after coronavirus, which may be a sign that the virus has caused kidney damage.

30. **Brain pressure:** The long-term extreme effects of COVID- 19 remain a mystery, but the survey found that 119 people who had the virus suffered from brain pressure. A study published in the Journal of the Brazilian Society of Tropical Medicine found a potential link between COVID-19 and benign intracranial hypertension, a condition that causes pressure in the brain. These symptoms are usually temporary but can be serious if they get worse and are left untreated.

31. **Swollen lymph nodes:** According to the Cleveland Clinic, swollen lymph nodes are usually a sign that your body is fighting an infection. Your glands are working hard to flush out toxins and cells through lymph fluid. When your body fights a virus like COVID-19, lymph nodes may swell as all hands are on deck trying to get rid of the illness.

32. **Head pressure:** One of the common symptoms of COVID- 19 is a headache, but 128 survey participants reported feel- ing extreme pressure at the base of their head or occipital nerve after recovering from the virus. According to the American Association of Neurological Surgeons, pressure at the occipital nerve (the nerves that run through the scalp) may be caused by muscle tightness or pinched nerves. These nerves may experience pressure or pain during an infection or due to blood vessel inflammation.

33. **Rashes:** According to a study published in JAMA Dermatology, the virus may be associated with a number of different skin rashes. The study found two different types of rashes that occurred in some patients infected with the coronavirus: the petechial flexural eruption and digitate papulosquamous rashes. These skin conditions could occur at any time during and after infection and may contribute to the feeling of burning skin.

34. **Body, joint, and bone aches** are common with coronavirus and most other illnesses. According to one study, when the immune system is in overdrive, it causes an immune response that ramps up your white blood cells and causes them to produce glycoproteins called interleukins. These can cause joint pain, bone pain, and swelling.

35. **Vessel irregularities:** These feelings of hot blood rushing may be due to blood vessel irregularities caused by the virus or remnants of a fever. According to a study published in *Science Daily*, this sudden rise in

temperature may be your immune system cranking up in an attempt to continue killing off the virus. The study found that "elevated body temperature helps certain types of immune cells to work better."

36. **Chills without a fever** was a long-lasting COVID-19 symptom for 154 survey participants. It could be the body's way of continuing to regulate temperature and recover from a previous fever. According to Keck Medicine of USC, chills without a fever may also indicate your body is under stress and fighting a viral or bacterial infection, or you're dealing with low blood sugar, which makes sense if you didn't eat much while you were sick.

37. **Neck pain:** According to John Hopkins Medicine, your neck doesn't have much protection or support, so neck pain is common. Since the virus is known to cause muscle and joint pain as well as body aches, your sensitive neck is more susceptible to this lingering symptom.

38. **Tongue pain and soreness:** According to the University of Florida Health, tongue pain and soreness can be caused by several factors, such as infection, hypothyroidism, or a tumor in the pituitary gland. A study published in the *International Journal of Infectious Diseases* found that oral mucosal lesions may be associated with COVID- 19 patients, which could explain this long-lasting virus symptom.

39. **Heat intolerance:** According to the CDC, one of the most common symptoms of COVID-19 is a fever. The body may need time after a fever has dissipated to recover and regu- late its temperature. This may be why 165 survey respondents claim to have heat intolerance after being infected with COVID-19. As the immune system fights off the virus, it raises and lowers the body's temperature accordingly, which may cause this heat intolerance to linger.

40. **Swollen hands and feet:** Those who contracted COVID- 19 and experienced "COVID toes" or other skin-related symptoms may also be dealing with swollen hands and feet. According to the Mayo Clinic, this welling is called edema, and it could be linked to kidney or heart problems, both of which may be caused by coronavirus.

41. **Dry skin may be attributed to the rashes** and cutaneous manifestations that some people developed on their skin due to the virus. However, according to the American Skin Association, dry skin

may also be attributed to a decline in fluid intake, which can happen when you're sick. It may also be a telling sign of a thyroid problem or hormonal imbalance.

42. **According to A&D Medical, "high blood pressure** is not a documented symptom of COVID-19, but it can exacerbate the symptoms of the virus." The 181 survey respondents who report experiencing high blood pressure after having COVID-19 likely already suffered from this condition, but fighting the virus may have made it worse.

43. **Living with a dry cough and sore throat:** According to the World Health Organization (WHO), COVID-19 symptoms generally include a dry cough and sore throat. Living with a dry cough and sore throat throughout the course of the virus may cause this dry throat to remain for a while, even after testing negative for COVID-19.

44. **Postnasal drip** is when mucus drips down the back of your throat, and it's common after you've had a stuffy or runny nose. After dealing with allergy or sinus issues or infections, postnasal drip can linger for a while. If one's body produced extra mucus and fluids to fight off the virus, this mucus might continue to drip. According to Harvard Health Publishing, you can treat postnasal drip by staying hydrated, taking a nasal decongestant, or inhaling steam, such as from a hot shower.

45. **Weight loss: COVID-19 survivors** who had severe cases are likely to experience extreme weight loss. According to an article posted by Northeast Ohio Medical University, it's common for patients who survive severe infections or illnesses to lose weight. When sufferers are placed on ventilators or hospitalized for long periods of time, their bodies don't obtain the proper nutrition or muscle-building exercise. The body is also under stress fighting off the virus, which can cause this weight loss to occur. COVID-19 survivors who had severe cases are likely to experience extreme weight loss. According to an article posted by Northeast Ohio Medical University, it's common for patients who survive severe infections or illnesses to lose weight. When sufferers are placed on ventilators or hospitalized for long periods of time, their bodies don't obtain the proper nutrition or muscle-building exercise.

The body is also under stress fighting off the virus, which can cause this weight loss to occur.

46. **Feeling irritable or angry:** According to MedPage Today, it's not uncommon for patients recovering from COVID- 19 to feel irritable or angry.

47. **Muscle twitches:** According to the University of Florida Health, muscle twitches may be caused by stress, lack of nutrients, or lack of sleep. Coronavirus is known to make its sufferers tired and their bodies stressed from fighting the virus, so this may explain muscle twitching. In some cases, it may be a sign of muscle damage or nervous system disorders.

48. **Mild confusion or "brain fog"** is a common symptom of coronavirus and most colds, flues, and viruses. According to an article published in *Science Magazine*, this confusion may occur because the body's systems are focused on fighting the illness, not giving enough focus, blood, or alertness to the brain.

49. **Lung pressure:** According to the CDC, persistent pressure or pain in the chest is a symptom of COVID-19, and 210 survey participants claim to continue feeling this symptom after the virus is gone. As a respiratory virus, it's possible that this pain or pressure is actually being felt in the lungs. However, according to Diagnostic and Interventional Cardiology, stroke, heart failure, arrhythmias, and other cardiac events have also been linked to coronavirus, so sufferers should take this lingering symptom seriously.

50. **Decrease in taste:** A loss of sense of taste is a common symptom of COVID-19, but 221 survey respondents claim the virus may have completely changed their sense of taste. According to Kaiser Permanente, a loss of sense of taste or partial loss may cause tastes to change. These changes may also be caused by a decrease in taste buds or changes in the way the nervous system processes certain taste sensations.

51. **Tinnitus is a ringing or noise in the ear,** and 233 survey respondents claim they now experience this ringing or humming in the ears after recovering from COVID-19. According to the American Tinnitus Association, the onset of tinnitus may occur due to stress and anxiety

after there's been damage to the inner ear, or when other conditions or diseases are developed.

52. **Neurological damage:** According to a study published in the Elsevier Public Health Emergency Collection, "viral infections have detrimental impacts on neurological functions, and even cause severe neurological damage." Two hundred forty-three survey participants reported feeling nerve sensations after COVID-19, which may be due to neurological damage caused by the virus.

53. **Constant thirst:** When you contract an illness or a virus like coronavirus, your body's working overtime to fight it. According to the Mayo Clinic, your body needs more fluids when you're sick, and if it doesn't get the fluids, you're likely to suffer from constant thirst. It's your body's way of telling you it's not getting enough fluids to continue fighting and recovering from the virus.

54. **Mucus membranes:** In some COVID-19 cases, patients have developed rashes on their skin. According to a research letter published in e *JAMA Network*, some coronavirus patients suffered from enanthcm, a skin rash that looks like small white spots on the mucous membranes. Other patients had widespread urticaria, or hives, on their skin. Other rashes were also found in some COVID-19 patients who were studied. Scientists aren't sure if this side effect is directly related to the virus or attributed to certain medications.

55. **Flashes of light:** According to UCLA Health, "floaters" are little specks or lines that float around in your field of vision every once a while. If you constantly see floaters, or they're accompanied by flashes of light, it may indicate you have a retina tear or vitreous detachment, which occurs when vitreous gel in the eye separates from the retina. In the survey, 249 respondents claimed to suffer from floaters or flashes of light in their vision after COVID-19.

56. **Back pain:** As with most illnesses, coronavirus is associated with muscle aches and pains. Patients with COVID-19 who were bedridden or spent an extended period inactive may experience upper back pain due to immobility. According to Kaiser Permanente, upper back pain isn't as common as lower back pain, but may be caused by muscle strain, poor posture, or pressure on the spinal nerves.

57. **Fatigue is a common symptom** of coronavirus, but some sufferers are having trouble shaking off that tiredness. According to an article published in the *Scientist*, it's possible that COVID-19 may lead to chronic illness, including chronic fatigue. Scientists are tracking these symptoms among sufferers who seek treatment, so they can get a grasp on what other symptoms may lead to chronic illness.

58. **Anxiety:** According to Northwestern Medicine, tremors may be caused by stress, anxiety, or too much caffeine. Tremors or shakes when you pick up a glass of water or hold a piece of paper may also indicate that you have essential tremor (ET), which is a neurological disorder that causes these shakes. These tremors may occur because the body is recovering from the stress of the virus, they may indicate ET, or there may be another underlying cause.

59. **Dehydration:** According to the University of Rochester Medical Center, muscle cramps usually occur after heavy exercise, when you're experiencing muscle fatigue, or if your body's dehydrated. Since the virus and other illnesses are notorious for dehydrating your body and causing muscle fatigue, these calf cramps may be an explainable symptom of coronavirus. Massaging, stretching, and warm compresses could help mitigate these cramps.

60. **Itchy, dry, and red eyes:** An article published in *Review of Optometry* reviewed the relationship between ocular symptoms and coronavirus in Chinese patients. It found that 27 percent of those studied complained of itchy, dry, and red eyes. Some even began to develop sore and dry eyes a few days before any other COVID-19 symptoms. Researchers feel this may be because coronavirus "infects the mucosa membrane epithelium and even lymphocytes, which are both abundant in ocular surface tissue."

61. **Ear pain, muffled hearing, or dizziness:** According to the Mayo Clinic, when your ears are clogged, "your eustachian tube which runs between your middle ear and the back of your nose—becomes obstructed." It may cause pressure, ear pain, muffled hearing, or dizziness. The survey found that 267 participants experienced clogged ears as a long-lasting symptom of COVID-19. Since clogged ears are common with a stuffy nose and other respiratory illnesses or sinus

infections, it's a common symptom of coronavirus. To relieve pressure, you can try popping your ears or taking a nasal decongestant.

62. **Nausea or vomiting:** While it's not usually listed as a common symptom of COVID-19, many who got the virus also suffered from nausea, vomiting, diarrhea, or other gastrointestinal problems. The survey found that 314 respondents claimed they still suffered from nausea or vomiting after coronavirus. According to the Mayo Clinic, these gastro-intestinal symptoms were varied, and some felt them well before a diagnosis. Others only dealt with these symptoms for one day.

63. **Shortness of breath** is a common symptom of COVID-19, but 318 survey participants reported that they continued to feel shortness of breath or exhaustion when they bent over. According to Penn Medicine, this may be a sign of an ongoing pulmonary problem or heart problem. While shortness of breath is common with COVID-19 sufferers, those who have recovered should seek medical attention if this symptom doesn't seem to be going away.

64. **Myalgia:** COVID-19 causes myalgia, pain in a muscle or a group of muscles. An article published in Nature Public Health Emergency Collection concludes that myalgia in COVID-19 patients lingers longer than it may with other illnesses. Lower back pain is usually associated with pneumonia or poor lung function, and since COVID-19 is a respiratory virus, it makes sense that patients are more likely to experience this type of muscle pain.

65. **Gastrointestinal issues:** While not a common symptom of COVID-19, many who contracted the virus did report gastrointestinal problems. This could explain why 344 survey respondents reported dealing with abdominal pain well after contracting the virus. In a study published through the American Gastrological Association, 31.9 percent of COVID-19 patients studied claimed to have gastrointestinal problems associated with the virus.

66. **While a dry cough is** most associated with coronavirus, some patients may experience phlegm in the back of their throat during the later stages. For coronavirus patients dealing with phlegm, the University of Maryland Medical System suggests taking an expectorant to help get the mucus out and make your cough more productive. Staying

hydrated and drinking warm beverages may also help to break up the phlegm.

67. **Loss of taste,** called ageusia, and loss of smell, called anosmia, are common symptoms of the virus, and the duration of these symptoms varies by patient. A study published in the *Journal of Korean Medical Science* analyzed Korean COVID-19 sufferers and the duration of this specific symptom. The study found that "most patients with anosmia or ageusia recovered within three weeks."

68. **Heartburn occurs** when stomach acid backs up into the tube that carries food from your mouth to your stomach (esophagus), according to the Mayo Clinic. Since the virus is known to cause gastrointestinal problems, some patients may take longer to recover from these inconsistencies than others. Avoiding alcohol, spicy foods, and large meals may help curb these long-lasting symptoms.

69. **Neuropathy is weakness or numbness due to nerve dam- age.** Since the virus can do some damage to the nervous system, this may be a lingering symptom for some sufferers. According to a report published in the *Elsevier Public Health Emergency Collection*, COVID-19 may even disguise itself as motor peripheral neuropathy without other symptoms. Nerve fibers may be more sensitive when a patient is infected with the virus, causing this numbing of the hands and feet.

70. **Sadness: As a pandemic,** COVID-19 sufferers are required to quarantine, which may mean isolating from loved ones and not being able to engage in activities they enjoy. A study published in the *Lancet* analyzed the mental side effects of the virus and concluded that medical professionals should watch their patients for signs of depression or some neuropsychiatric syndromes well after recovery.

71. **Congested or runny nose:** According to the American Pharmacists Association, the CDC recently added "runny nose" as a symptom of COVID-19. Four hundred fourteen survey respondents claimed a congested or runny nose as a lingering symptom of the virus. A runny nose is one way to get rid of the mucus in your body after the virus, so it may persist until the mucus is gone.

72. **Blurry vision** may be a sign of nerve damage or may also occur when other COVID-19 symptoms are going strong, such as a fever or

headache. According to the American Academy of Ophthalmology, blurred vision may also be a symptom of endophthalmitis, which is an infection of tissue or fluids inside the eye. If this is the case, quick treatment is required to prevent blindness.

73. **Hair loss:** According to Dr. Shilpi Harpal MD, from the Cleveland Clinic, hair loss isn't necessarily a symptom of COVID-19, but maybe a side effect of the virus. She states, "We are seeing patients who had COVID-19 two to three months ago and are now experiencing hair loss." In the survey, 423 respondents reported experiencing hair loss after the coronavirus. Dr. Khetarpal says this may be due to a change in diet, high fever, extreme weight loss, or any other "shock to the system" that COVID-19 may have caused.

74. **Chills:** The CDC conducted a study on coronavirus patients and found that 96 percent of patients recovered from chills, and 97 percent recovered from fever. While most recovered from all COVID-19 symptoms, 34 percent still revealed that they were suffering from one or more lasting symptoms when interviewed four to eight days after testing positive. Sixty-five percent of sufferers returned to their usual state of health around seven days after testing positive, but chronic medical conditions, age, weight, gender, and other factors may affect how long symptoms— such as fever and chills—last.

75. **Tachycardia:** According to the Mayo Clinic, tachycardia occurs when your heart beats over one hundred beats per minute. It's a form of arrhythmia, or a heartbeat disorder. In the survey, 448 respondents experienced tachycardia after suffering from COVID-19. It may be the body's response to stress, trauma, or illness. However, if tachycardia is left untreated and continues to occur, it can lead to serious complications, such as heart failure or stroke.

76. **Partial or complete loss of sense of smell** is a common symptom of COVID-19 and many other respiratory viruses, according to Penn Medicine. Since your olfactory system is so close to your respiratory system, virus cells can enter nerve and receptor cells and cause damage. It can take a long time for these cells to repair, and some cells may never fully recover from the virus.

77. **Night sweats:** According to Kaiser Permanente, night sweats are different from regular sweating because they occur only at night and include intense sweating, enough to soak through your clothes and sheets. It's possible that night sweats are present due to a residual fever, but they may also be caused by thyroid level issues, menopause, anxiety, or infections. New medication or other lingering symptoms, such as chills and muscle aches, may also contribute to long-lasting night sweats.

78. **Sore throat:** While not all coronavirus sufferers experience a sore throat, it's one of the common symptoms the CDC lists for the virus. According to the CDC, viruses and infections cause sore throats, which may be why this is a linger- ing symptom for some coronavirus patients.

79. **Diarrhea:** While it's not the most common, diarrhea is listed by the CDC as a symptom of COVID-19. A study conducted by several researchers analyzed 206 patients with low severity COVID-19, and 48 experienced digestive problems first before other coronavirus symptoms. Diarrhea lasted an average of fourteen days for COVID-19 patients in the study.

80. **Heart palpitations:** Even after the fever, headache, and dry cough have disappeared, some patients who have "recovered" from COVID-19 may experience heart palpitations. A study published in JAMA Cardiology examined one hundred recovered COVID-19 patients and found that seventy-eight of them had "cardiac involvement" while 60 percent had ongoing myocardial inflammation. Ongoing heart issues, such as palpitations, may be long-lasting for COVID-19 patients regardless of their illness severity.

81. **Joint pain:** Dr. Richard Deem from Cedars-Sinai explains that as your immune system attempts to fight off COVID- 19 or any type of illness, white blood cells produce interleukins to help join the fight. While these interleukins are useful in fighting off the virus cells, they also cause muscle and joint pain. The immune response may still be heightened in these recovering patients, causing this joint pain to last.

82. **Cough:** A lingering cough can be a side effect of any type of cold, flu, or illness. According to a study conducted by the World Health

Organization (WHO) on Chinese COVID-19 patients, 61.7 percent developed a dry cough. As a respiratory virus, the cough associated with COVID-19 may take a long time to go away because your body is attempting to get rid of lingering mucus and phlegm.

83. **Persistent chest pain or pressure:** Chest pain or pressure was a common lingering COVID-19 symptom among survey participants. Since coronavirus affects the lungs and respiratory system, this chest pain may be attributed to the virus still settling in the body. According to the Mayo Clinic, sudden, sharp chest pains are referred to as pleurisy, and it may indicate that the lung walls are inflamed. Pleurisy may be a sign of pneumonia or another type of infection, so recovered COVID-19 patients should see a doctor if this symptom persists.

84. **Dizziness:** COVID-19 is a respiratory virus that also has nervous system side effects. According to a study published in the *Journal of the American College of Emergency Physicians Open*, "symptoms including headache, dizziness, vertigo, and paresthesia have been reported." This may be due to decreased oxygen levels, dehydration, fevers, or headaches also caused by the virus.

85. **Memory problems:** A paper published in the *Journal of Alzheimer's Disease* analyzes potential long-term neurological effects of COVID-19 on patients who experienced severe cases. Memory problems and cognitive decline are potential side effects for some of these patients. Since the virus affects the nervous system, memory problems may be a lingering side effect for some patients, especially those who have suffered severe cases.

86. **Anxiety:** According to a poll conducted by the American Psychiatric Association, about 36 percent of Americans feel coronavirus has had a serious impact on their mental health. Between quarantining, social isolation, and worry about developing a severe case of coronavirus, it's no wonder anxiety is a lingering symptom for COVID-19 patients.

87. **Difficulty sleeping:** Sleep is crucial because it keeps the immune system functioning properly, heightens brain function, stabilizes mood, and improves mental health. Seven hundred eighty-two survey respondents claimed they were having difficulty sleeping even after recovering from COVID-19. This lack of sleep may be due to anxiety or

worry about the virus or may be attributed to other lingering symptoms, such as muscle pain or cough. Setting specific bedtimes and only using your bed for sleep may help with these difficulties.

88. **Headache:** According to Dr. Sandhya Mela with the Hartford HealthCare Headache Center, "it is estimated that headache is a symptom of COVID-19 in about 13 percent of patients with COVID-19." It is the fifth most common COVID-19 symptom after fever, cough, muscle aches, and trouble breathing." In the survey, 902 participants claimed that a headache was a long-lasting symptom after COVID-19. This may be due to dehydration, congestion, or other symptoms of coronavirus, such as a fever.

89. **Inability to exercise or be active:** After recovering from COVID-19, some patients find it hard to exercise or be active, even if they were fit before contracting the virus. Nine hundred sixteen survey participants reported that they were still unable to exercise after recovering from coronavirus. According to a study published in *JAMA Cardiology*, researchers recommend that patients who suffered from severe cases of COVID-19 wait at least two weeks before resuming light exercise. This allows time for doctors to see if heart or lung conditions develop that could make it dangerous to engage in physical activity.

90. **Difficulty concentrating or focusing:** The long-term effects of COVID-19 are unknown since the virus is so new, but researchers are seeing certain neurological effects on patients who have recovered. Studies conducted in Wuhan analyzed these neurological conditions and found that 40 percent of the patients analyzed experienced confusion and conscious disturbance. This is commonly referred to as "brain fog," and many patients express feeling this way while recovering from coronavirus.

91. **Muscle or body aches:** Body aches are a common symptom of many illnesses, including coronavirus. In this survey, 1,048 participants reported feeling these body aches after their COVID-19 diagnosis. According to Dr. Tania Elliott, MD FAAAAI, FACAAI, "Your body aches when you have the flu because your immune system is revving up to fight infection." It's not necessarily the virus that causes these aches but your body's own reaction to the virus invasion.

92. **Fatigue was the most common lingering symptom of coronavirus.**
According to a study conducted by the WHO, the average recovery
time for mild coronavirus cases is around two weeks, but three to six
weeks for severe or critical cases. Lingering fatigue may be a sign that
your body is still fighting the virus.

# ABOUT THE AUTHOR

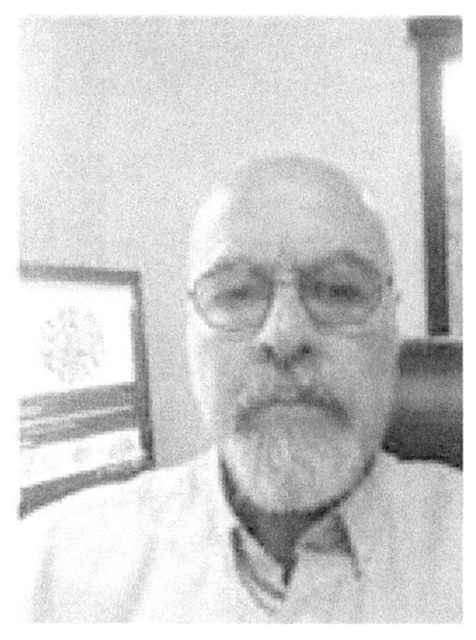

Frank Hamo, PhD in biomedical engineering, is the founder and CEO of MTI. He spent his entire biomedical engineering career bridging the gap of medicine and engineering to deliver advanced healthcare monitoring options. His mission is to utilize latest biomedical engineering technology to improve early detection, monitoring, and screening devices, improve operational efficiency of healthcare organizations to save billions of dollars in medical treatment, replace current medical screening methods, and actualize portable at-home devices.

He had lost seven members of his family for cancer therefore he spent numbers of years looking at cancer research because he believes understanding the disease and how to approach and manage it on time can increase chances of survivor and recovery, he comes to conclusion that early prediction, early signs and detection of cancer can cure it at early stages before losing control; at the same time he believes cancer cells can be defeated by understanding how the immune system attacks foreign antigen.

Also, for the last two years, since COVID-19 emerged as global pandemic, Hamo has been tracking the virus mutation from day one and providing recommendations for diagnosis, symptoms managements to assist physicians and health workers to distinguish between COVID-19 related illness, preexisting chronical conditions or as long hauler post-COVID-19 illnesses. Also identified if COVID 19 infection can awaken cancer cells.

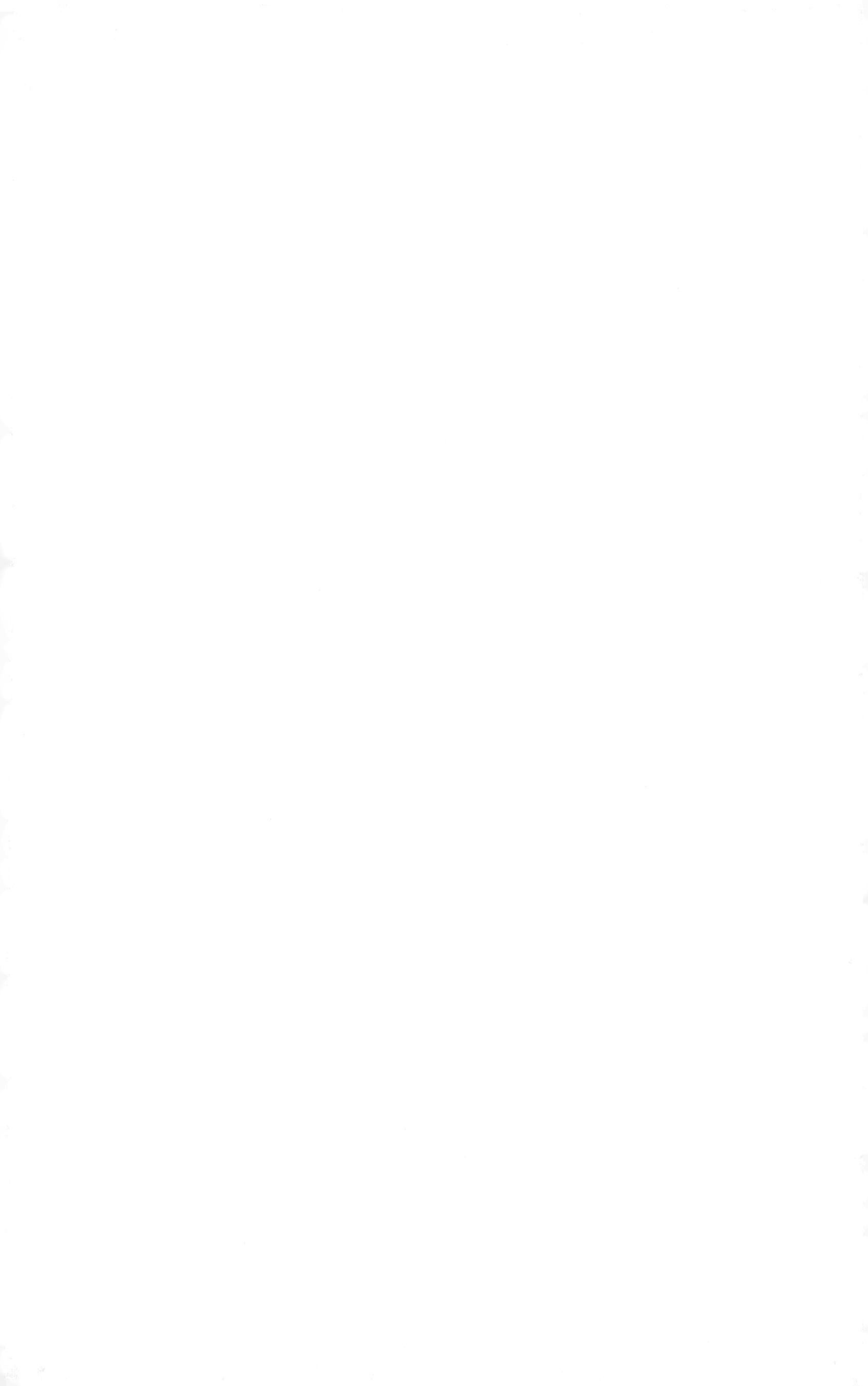

www.ingramcontent.com/pod-product-compliance
Lightning Source LLC
Chambersburg PA
CBHW061538120726
48001CB00004B/1611